Pregnancy Countdown
a day-by-day guide to waiting for baby

Pregnancy Countdown

a day-by-day guide to waiting for baby

Paula Ford-Martin

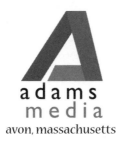

adams
media
avon, massachusetts

First published in the US in 2005 ISBN 1-59337-510-7

Published by Adams Media
Adams Media is an F+W Publications Inc. Company
57 Littlefield Street, Avon, MA 02322
1-800-872-5627

J I H G F E D C B A

Printed in the USA by Maple-Vail

Visit our website at www.adamsmedia.com

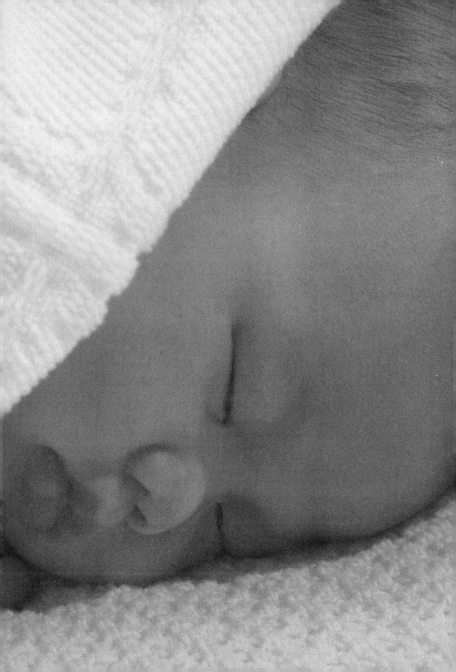

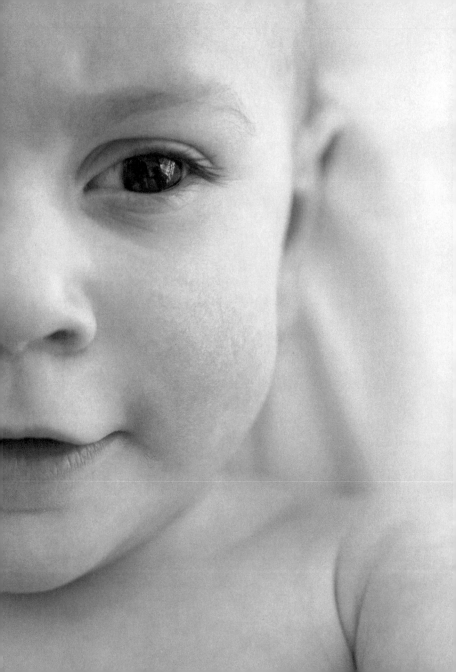

Pregnancy Countdown is a unique countdown calendar to your pregnancy. Based on the pregnancy term, not the calendar year, this book provides a day-by-day guide to your own personal experience of waiting for baby.

Starting from the month in which you become pregnant and running up to your calculated due date, this beautifully illustrated guide is packed full of information on the physical and emotional changes experienced in pregnancy; a week-by-week guide to your developing baby; hints and tips on health and fitness; plus vital information on childbirth and how to best prepare for your labor.

In addition there are facts, reminders, warnings and your questions answered on every aspect of pregnancy, labor and parenting skills. Plus a selection of baby names to choose from and fun quotes from well-known celebrities on the joys of parenthood.

Pregnancy Countdown offers nuggets of information day-by-day for the busy mom-to-be. It also provides an opportunity for you to record your thoughts and feelings during this very precious period of your life—to make a record that you, and your child, can treasure for a lifetime.

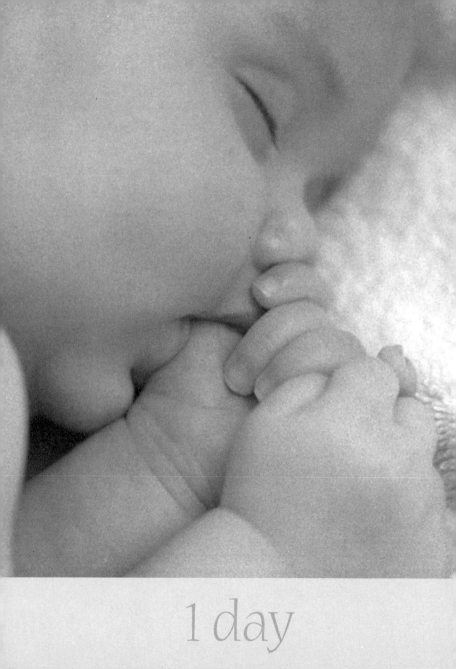

1 day

day 1

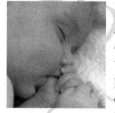

Did You Know?

After sexual intercourse the sperm cells work their way through the womb towards the Fallopian tube. The sperm cell penetrates the ovum: the tail of the sperm cell lets go and only the head melts together with the core of the ovum. On completion of this process—which takes about half an hour—all the genetic characteristics of your new baby have been determined.

Thoughts and Feelings...

....
....
....
....
....
....
....
....
....
....

reminder

A good intake of folic acid helps prevent neural tube defects, such as spina bifida, in the developing baby. Take folic acid as soon as you start trying for a baby or at least during the first 12 weeks of pregnancy.

DIARY DATES: ....
....

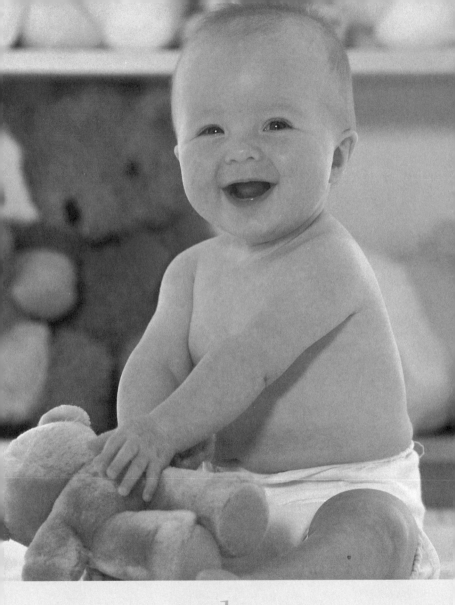

2 days

day 2

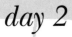

Giving Birth

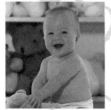

Most births happen within the period running two weeks before to two weeks after your calculated due date (see How to calculate your due date). A pregnancy normally lasts 266 days, or 38 weeks (40 weeks calculated from the first day of the last period). Almost 10 percent of pregnancies last 40 weeks—two weeks over the calculated date—only 5 percent last 41 weeks—three weeks over the calculated date—and less than 1% of the babies arrive four weeks 'overdue'.

Thoughts and Feelings...

....

....

....

....

....

....

....

tip · tip ·

IF THIS IS YOUR FIRST PREGNANCY YOU ARE MORE LIKELY TO GO PAST YOUR DUE DATE. IF YOU HAVE GIVEN BIRTH BEFORE, HOWEVER, YOU WILL PROBABLY GIVE BIRTH WITHIN FOUR DAYS OF YOUR CALCULATED DUE DATE.

DIARY DATES: ....

....

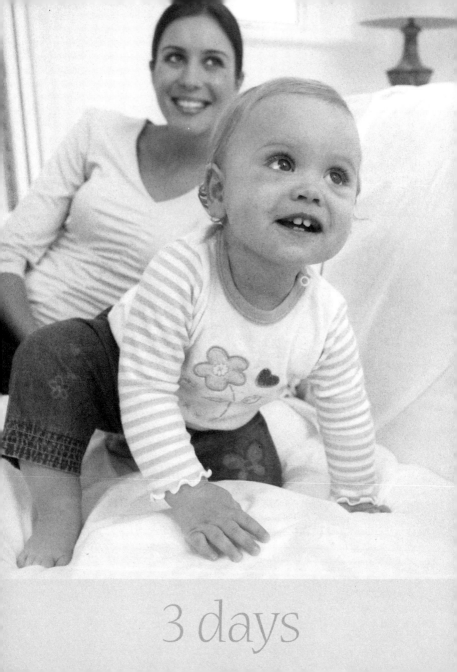

3 days

day 3

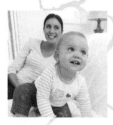

Health and Fitness

A pregnant woman is not expected to gain too much weight during the course of her pregnancy. However, this is not the time to go on a diet as restricting what you eat could create shortages for you or the baby. Eating properly during pregnancy does not mean eating for two, but really thinking about what you eat and trying to eat twice as healthily.

Thoughts and Feelings...

....
....
....
....
....
....
....
....
....

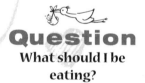

Question
What should I be eating?

· *Plenty of fresh fruit and vegetables*

· *Plenty of fiber to combat constipation*

· *Avoid unpasteurized dairy products, variety meats (liver, kidneys, tongue etc.), and undercooked eggs, meat, poultry and pâtés.*

· *Limit your caffeine intake*

· *Give in to your cravings—but don't overdo it*

DIARY DATES: ....

....

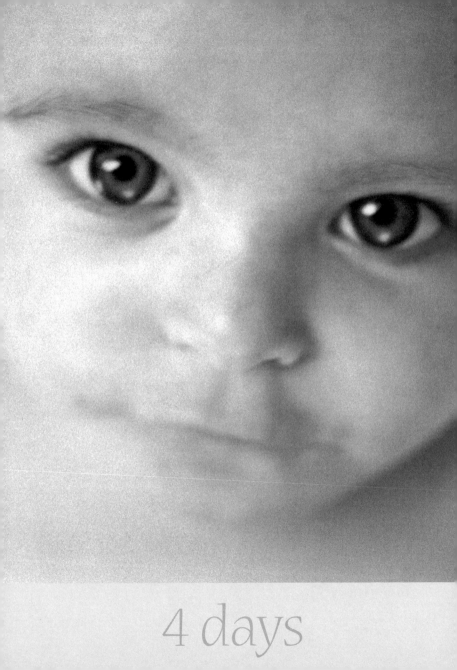

4 days

day 4

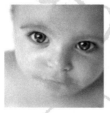

Baby's Development

In the first half of your menstrual cycle your body produces two hormones that are essential if you are to achieve a pregnancy. The first hormone stimulates the process that results, at ovulation, in the production of an egg. The second prepares the womb for the arrival of a fertilized ovum by stimulating the lining of the womb, called the endometrium, to thicken.

Thoughts and Feelings...

....
....
....
....
....
....
....
....
....
....
....

WARNING

AVOID MEDICATION WHENEVER POSSIBLE AS IT CAN UPSET THE DELICATE BALANCE OF CHEMICALS NEEDED IN THE BODY FOR SUCCESSFUL FERTILIZATION AND THE EARLY DEVELOPMENT OF THE BABY. IF YOU ARE ON LONG-TERM MEDICATION, TALK TO YOUR DOCTOR ABOUT YOUR OPTIONS BEFORE YOU GET PREGNANT.

DIARY DATES: ....
....

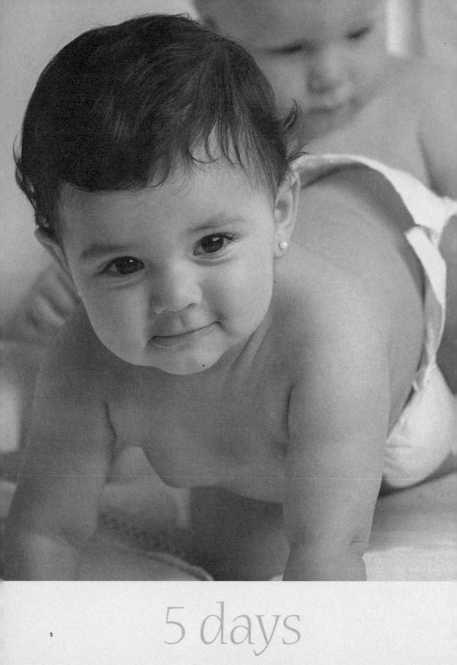

5 days

day 5

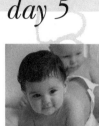

Did You Know?

It is never too soon to start thinking about what kind of delivery you would like. Hospital procedures can vary dramatically—start investigating what is available and talk your options through with your caregiver as soon as possible. If you are considering a home birth, ask your caregiver if doing so is allowed where you live and, if so, what regulations there may be.

"My heroes are and were my parents. I can't see having anyone else as my heroes."

Michael Jordan, basketball player

Thoughts and Feelings...

....

....

....

....

....

....

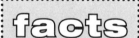

Your doctor will enquire about the family medical history of you and your baby's father. If there is a history of chronic illness or medical disorders you will be advised of the screening tests you may want to consider.

DIARY DATES: ....

....

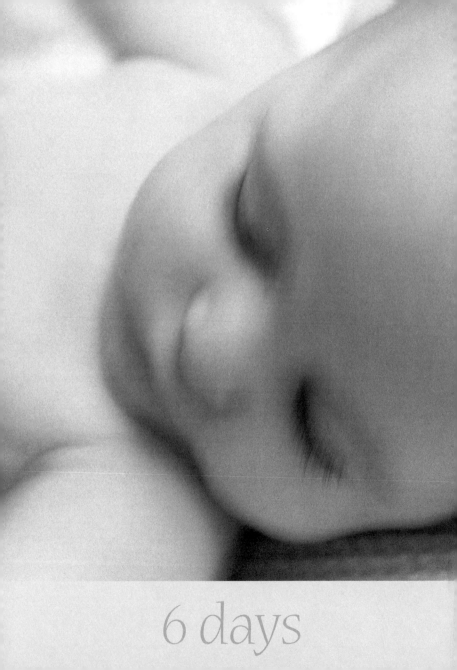

6 days

day 6

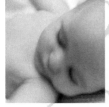

Baby Names for Girls

Abigail (Hebrew)	Amber (English)
Agnes (Greek)	Ambrosine (Greek)
Aidan (Irish)	Amelia (English)
Alexandra (Greek)	Andrea (Scottish)
Alice (English	Annabelle (English)
Alison (German)	Anne (English)
Amanda (Latin)	

Thoughts and Feelings…

....
....
....
....
....
....
....
....
....
....

IF YOU AND YOUR PARTNER ARE HAVING PROBLEMS AGREEING ON A NAME, ONE WAY TO PROCEED IS TO EACH DRAW UP A LIST. KEEP MAKING LISTS UNTIL YOU HIT ON A NAME THAT APPEARS ON BOTH LISTS AND THAT YOU BOTH LIKE.

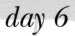

DIARY DAT: ....

....

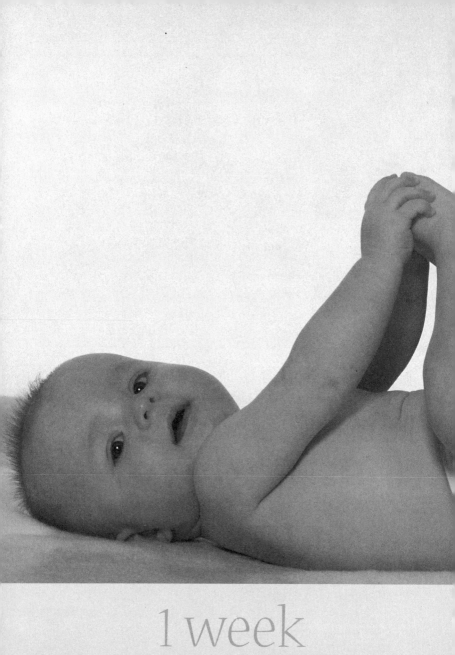

1 week

day 7

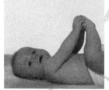

Your Pregnancy

From the moment of impregnation the pregnancy lasts 38 weeks on average. Generally speaking, the first day of your last period is counted as the first day of your pregnancy: the day that comes precisely 40 weeks after that will be your calculated due date (see How to calculate your due date). Slight confusion may arise if you have very erratic periods and if you are totally unable to remember when your last period started.

Thoughts and Feelings...

....
....
....
....
....
....
....
....
....

Question

I'm 40: what are my chances of an uncomplicated pregnancy?

Women over 35 have a higher chance of developing high blood pressure, diabetes or placental problems during pregnancy. The baby also has increased risk of Down's Syndrome in older mothers. However, good care during pregnancy can reduce both risks substantially.

DIARY DATES: ....

....

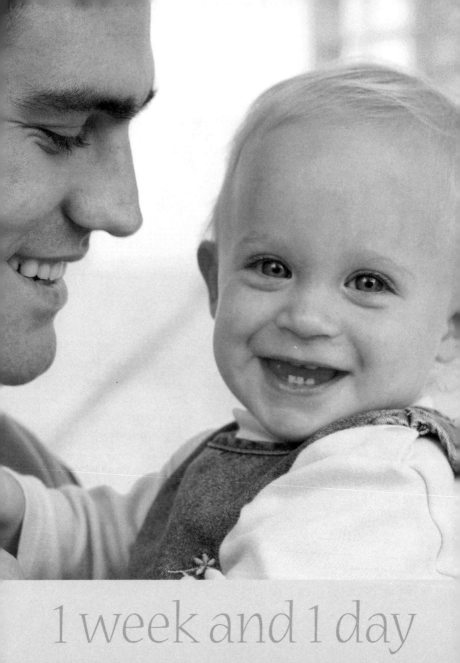

1 week and 1 day

day 8

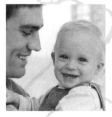

Did You Know?

For every 100 girls, 106 boys are born. So, statistically the chance of a boy is 51.5 percent and the chance of a girl is 48.5 percent. One, unproven, theory is that the female embryo is more at risk during the early stages of pregnancy. Another argument is that, over time, evolution provided more boys because, historically, their life was more dangerous and likely to end violently and early.

Thoughts and Feelings...

....
....
....
....
....
....
....
....
....
....

tip · tip

BREASTFEEDING IS GOOD FOR YOU AND GOOD FOR YOUR BABY. THE AVAILABILITY OF FORMULA MILK HAS PROVIDED AN ALTERNATIVE TO A FEEDING SYSTEM THAT IS AS OLD AS HUMANKIND ITSELF, BUT REMEMBER THIS: NUTRITIONALLY, BREAST MILK PROVIDES EVERYTHING YOUR BABY NEEDS.

DIARY DATES: ....

....

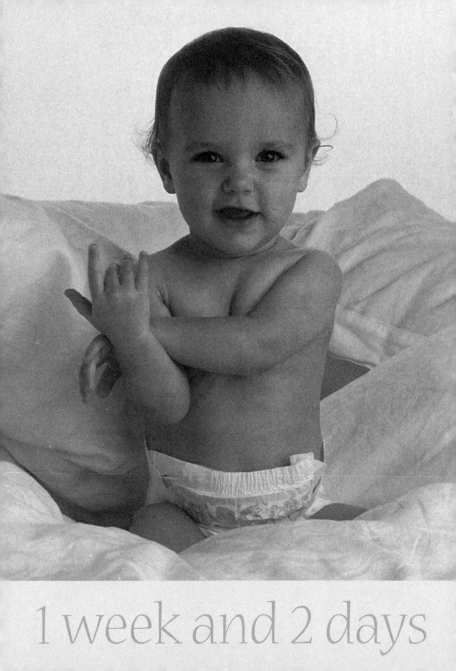

1 week and 2 days

day 9

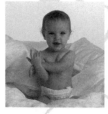

Giving Birth

If this is your first baby you may be concerned that you won't recognize the onset of labour and won't get to the hospital in time. You do hear spectacular stories of babies born in the back of taxis but this really is the exception rather than the rule. Labour lasts, on average, from 12 to 14 hours and you should have plenty of warning signs.

Thoughts and Feelings...

....
....
....
....
....
....
....
....
....
....

tip · tip

IF YOU ARE WORRIED ABOUT GETTING TO THE HOSPITAL ON TIME WORK OUT A ROUTE IN ADVANCE. KEEP THE CAR FILLED UP WITH GAS AND HAVE CASH AND A TELEPHONE NUMBER HANDY FOR A TAXI JUST IN CASE YOU NEED IT.

DIARY DATES: ....

....

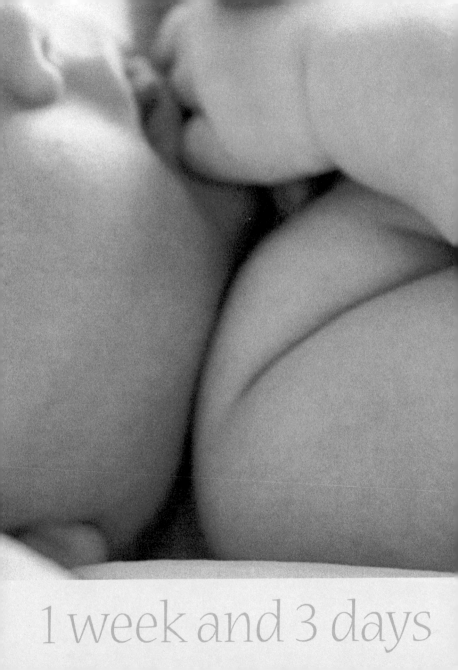

1 week and 3 days

day 10

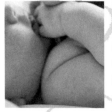

Health and Fitness

There is no need to gain any weight during the first trimester. The average weight gain throughout pregnancy is roughly 22–30lb (10–14kg). Slender women and women expecting multiples may be encouraged to gain a little more weight; women who are already overweight at the start of their pregnancy may be advised by their care provider to gain slightly less.

Thoughts and Feelings...

....

....

....

....

....

....

....

....

....

reminder

You only need an extra 300 calories a day during pregnancy. A glass of milk and a snack is probably enough—and milk provides calcium, which is great for baby.

DIARY DATES: ....

....

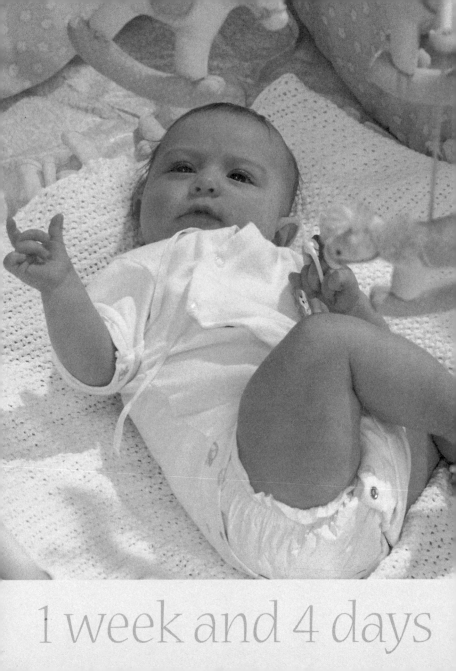

1 week and 4 days

day 11

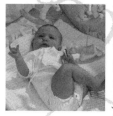

Baby's Development

The newly fertilized ovum is called a zygote. Your body sees to it—via small muscles in the Fallopian tubes—that the zygote is transported to the uterus (or womb). This journey takes three to four days, and during the trip the zygote has begun a process of rapid cell division. By the time the zygote reaches the uterus, it consists of a cluster of cells now known as a morula.

Thoughts and Feelings...

....
....
....
....
....
....
....
....
....

WARNING

PREGNANCY IS A STRESSFUL TIME. IF YOU ARE FEELING PARTICULARLY DOWN YOU MAY BE EXPERIENCING PRENATAL DEPRESSION. THIS COULD IMPACT ON YOUR DEVELOPING BABY AS WELL AS MAKING LIFE VERY TOUGH FOR YOU. DON'T WAIT—TALK TO YOUR CARE PROVIDER NOW.

DIARY DATES: ....
....

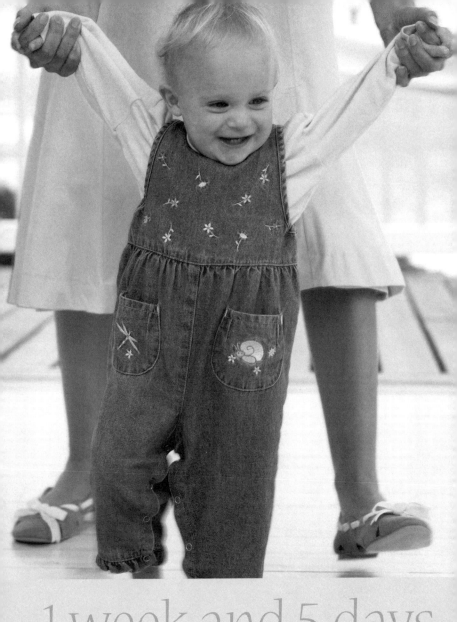

1 week and 5 days

day 12

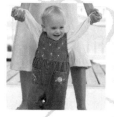

Did You Know?

Kids are remarkably adaptable. You may feel like your home is going to be turned upside down by the arrival of a baby, but remember that a child can thrive just about anywhere as long as it is given a healthy and nurturing environment. Think about setting up a changing area in the baby's bedroom—if you have space to give him one—and another downstairs, if you live in a house with stairs.

WARNING

IT IS ALSO IMPORTANT THAT BABIES HAVE A SAFE SPACE TO EXPLORE AND DEVELOP IN. MAKE SURE IT IS WELL VENTILATED AND INSULATED. CHECK FOR HAZARDS SUCH AS PEELING PAINT, SPLINTERS, BLIND CORDS AND ANY SMALL OBJECTS. AS SOON AS BABY ARRIVES, YOU WILL NOTICE A HUNDRED MORE DANGERS!

"You cannot catch a child's spirit by running after it; you must stand still and for love it will soon itself return."

Arthur Miller, playwright (1915–2005)

Thoughts and Feelings...

....

....

....

....

....

....

DIARY DATES: ....

....

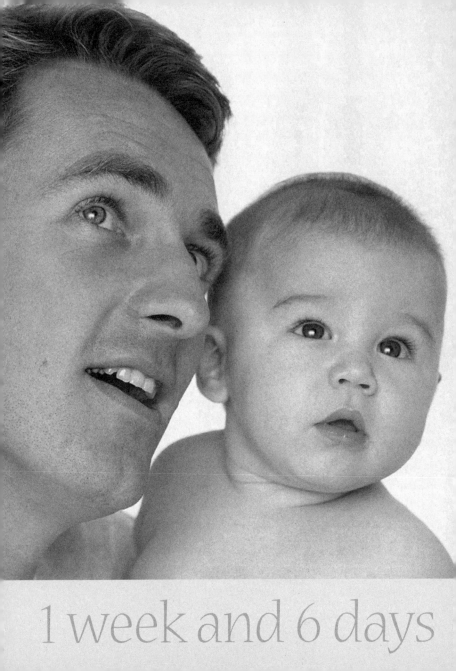

1 week and 6 days

day 13

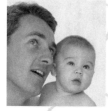

Baby Names for Boys

Aaron (Hebrew)
Adam (Hebrew)
Aidan (Irish)
Alan (English)
Alexander (Greek)
Andrew (English)

Angus (Scottish)
Anthony (Latin)
Arnold (German)
Arthur (Celtic)
Ashley (English)

Thoughts and Feelings...

....
....
....
....
....
....
....
....
....

tip · tip

IF YOU CAN'T DECIDE ON A TRADITIONAL BABY NAME, IT IS BECOMING INCREASINGLY COMMON TO ADOPT A NAME FROM ANOTHER SOURCE SUCH AS A PLANT, A COUNTRY, A COUNTY OR STATE, OR EVEN A CITY.

DIARY DATES: ....
....

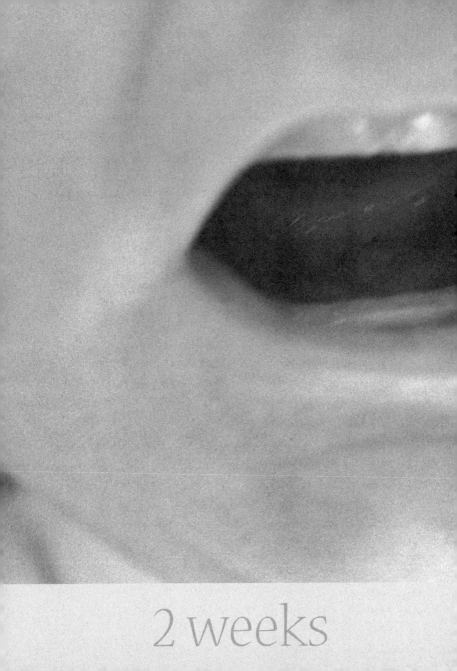

2 weeks

day 14

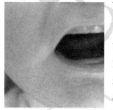

Your Pregnancy

If you are planning a pregnancy and wish to increase the chances of getting pregnant in a particular month, you can plan to have sexual intercourse around the time of ovulation. The egg takes 12 to 24 hours to travel down the Fallopian tubes. Ovulation prediction kits can now be bought at a pharmacy or you can keep a record of your temperature as a guide to ovulation.

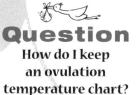

Question

How do I keep an ovulation temperature chart?

Check your body temperature daily before getting out of bed, starting on the first day of your period. A small rise will occur on the days after ovulation. If you do the test over two to three months you may find you always ovulate on a certain day.

Thoughts and Feelings...

....

....

....

....

....

....

....

....

....

DIARY DATES: ....

....

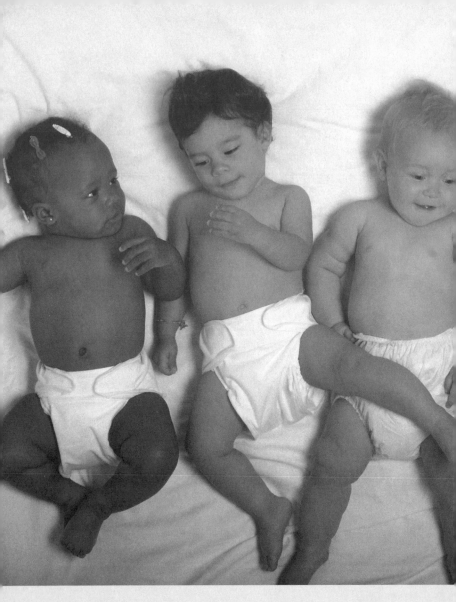

2 weeks and 1 day

day 15

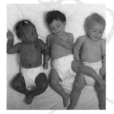

Did You Know?

The fertilized ovum has 23 pairs of chromosomes: the last pair of chromosomes is responsible for the sexual characteristics. The mother always supplies the X-chromosome. If the sperm cell from the father also has an X-chromosome in it, a girl will be born; if the father supplies a Y-chromosome, a boy will be born. It is therefore the father who determines the sex.

Thoughts and Feelings...

....

....

....

....

....

....

....

....

tip · tip

YOUR BABY'S DEVELOPMENT IS DETERMINED BY THE 46 CHROMOSOMES INHERITED FROM YOU (THE MOTHER), AND THE FATHER. CERTAIN GENETIC TESTS CAN REVEAL IF YOU ARE 'CARRIERS' OF CERTAIN CONDITIONS THAT COULD BE PASSED ON TO YOUR CHILD.

DIARY DATES: ....

....

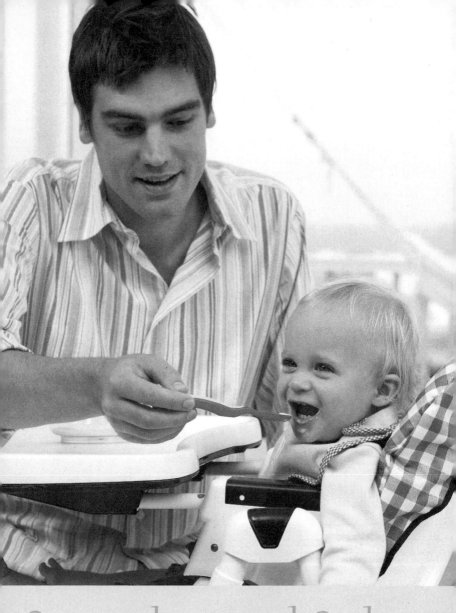

2 weeks and 2 days

day 16

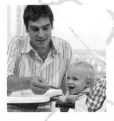

Giving Birth

Giving birth can be divided into three phases. The first phase is the dilation of the cervix, the second phase is the pushing out of the baby, and the third phase is the birth of the placenta. For most women, the stiffest challenge is faced during the first phase, which starts with the earliest signs of labor and lasts until the baby descends into the birth canal ready to be pushed out.

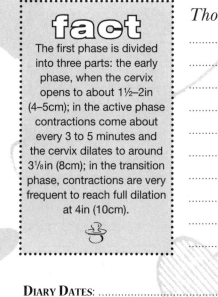

fact

The first phase is divided into three parts: the early phase, when the cervix opens to about 1½–2in (4–5cm); in the active phase contractions come about every 3 to 5 minutes and the cervix dilates to around 3⅛in (8cm); in the transition phase, contractions are very frequent to reach full dilation at 4in (10cm).

Thoughts and Feelings...

....

....

....

....

....

....

....

....

....

....

DIARY DATES: ....

....

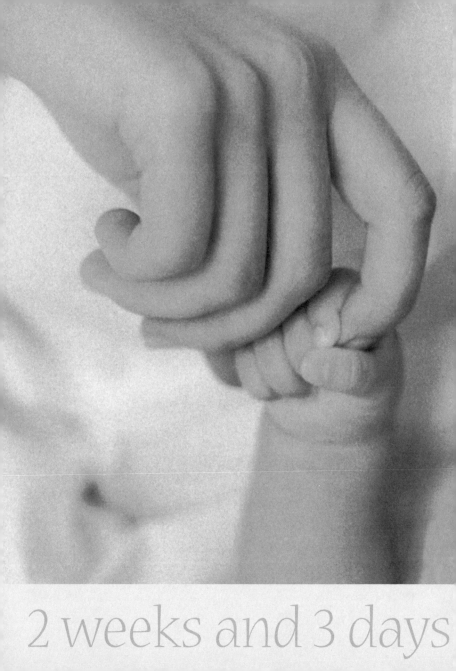

2 weeks and 3 days

day 17

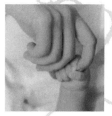

Health and Fitness

According to a survey of women in the United States, a pregnant woman takes, on average, 11 different medicines between fertilization and the time that the delivery begins; during the delivery itself she receives another seven. Taking medicines is always a question of weighing the pros and cons and following the advice of your care provider. Restrict the use of medicine to a minimum.

Thoughts and Feelings...

....
....
....
....
....
....
....
....
....
....

WARNING

BE WARY OF USING NATURAL REMEDIES TO TREAT MINOR AILMENTS SUCH AS COLDS. SUPPLEMENTS AND HERBAL TREATMENTS CAN BE POWERFUL MEDICINAL SUBSTANCES. ALWAYS CHECK WITH YOUR CARE PROVIDER BEFORE USING ALTERNATIVE MEDICINES DURING PREGNANCY.

DIARY DATES: ....
....

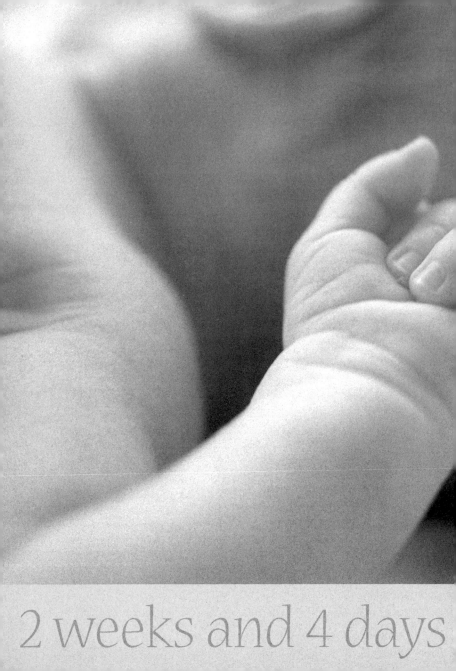

2 weeks and 4 days

day 18

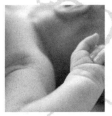

Baby's Development

The newly fertilized ovum is continuing its rapid cell division. Five or six days after fertilization, the zygote reaches the uterus (or womb) and becomes known as the blastocyst. It starts the process of implantation roughly one week after conception, as wispy fingers of tissues called the chorionic villi reach out to secure the blastocyst to the nutrient-rich wall of your uterus.

Thoughts and Feelings...

....

....

....

....

....

....

....

....

fact

Some women experience 'spotting,' very light vaginal bleeding, as the embryo implants itself. It will probably only last for one to two days and may be accompanied by gentle cramps. Coming 7 to 10 days after ovulation it may be mistaken for the start of menstruation.

Diary Dates: ....

....

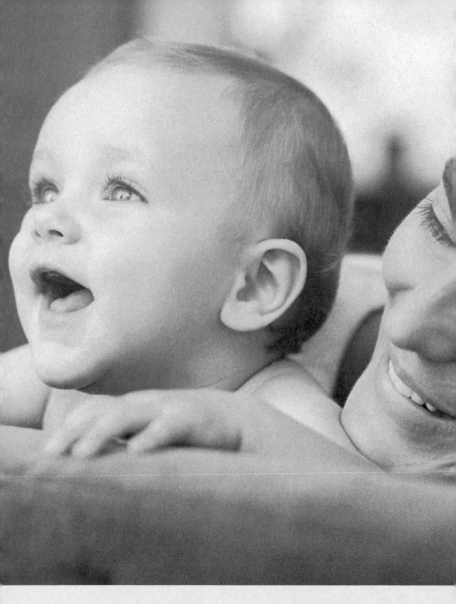

2 weeks and 5 days

day 19

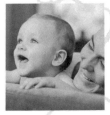

Did You Know?

About 17 in 20 couples conceive within a year of trying to get pregnant. About 19 in 20 couples conceive within two years. Generally it is worth talking to your doctor if you have not conceived after one year of trying—perhaps slightly sooner if you are over 35.

Thoughts and Feelings...

....

....

....

....

....

....

....

....

....

....

"Famous mothers long for a child for the same reasons as normal mothers. People usually only see your exterior but being rich, beautiful and famous can't stop you from feeling emptiness. You don't want a new role then, you want a baby."

Rene Russo, actress

(taken from *Beau Monde*)

DIARY DATES: ....

....

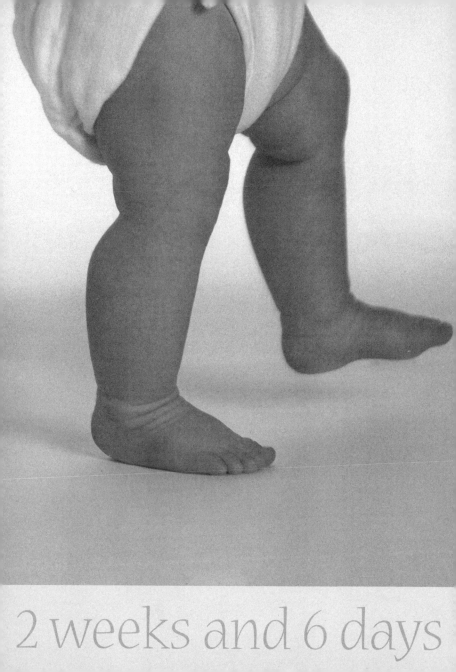

2 weeks and 6 days

2 weeks and 6 days

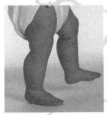

Baby Names for Girls

Barbara (Greek)   Beverly (English)
Bernadette (Frer.ch)   Billie (English)
Bernice (Greek)   Bonnie (English)
Bertha (German)   Brenda (English)
Beryl (Greek)   Bridget (Irish)
Bethany (English)   Bryony (English)

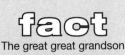

The great great grandson of Carlos III of Spain, don Alfonso de Borbón y Borbón (1866–1934), had 94 given names, several of which were double names. John and Margaret Nelson gave their daughter Tracey (born December 31, 1985) a total of 140 given names. *(Guinness Book of Records)*

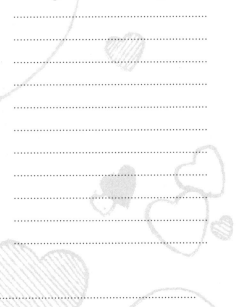

Thoughts and Feelings...

....
....
....
....
....
....
....
....
....
....
....

DIARY DATES: ....
....

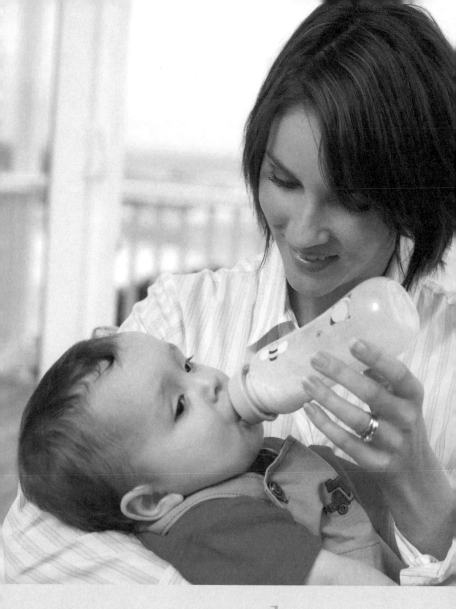

3 weeks

day 21

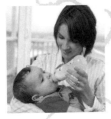

Your Pregnancy

Although fertilization has just taken place, the official pregnancy count already shows the third week: remember day one of your pregnancy is counted as the first day of your last menstrual period. Some women are extremely sensitive to hormonal changes; they may experience mood swings, swelling of the breasts with tenderness, and bloating just a few days after fertilization.

Thoughts and Feelings...

....
....
....
....
....
....
....
....
....
....

fact

Increased vaginal secretions are another hormonal side effect, and will continue throughout your pregnancy. They should be colorless, mucus like and odor- and pain-free. If this changes, consult your care provider as soon as possible to rule out infection.

DIARY DATES: ....
....

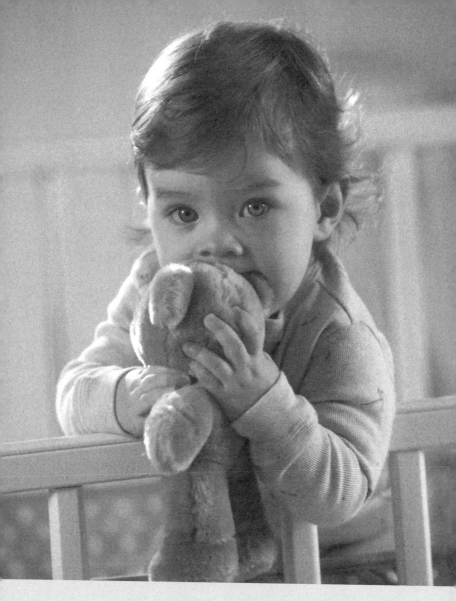

3 weeks and 1 day

day 22

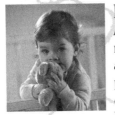

Did You Know?

At birth a baby girl already has about one million ova (eggs) in stock and no new ova are added to that. By the time she reaches puberty there are only 200,000 to 400,000 of them left. Still, this is more than enough, because each month only one ovum is released. On rare occasions two ova are released, which may result in fraternal (non-identical) twins.

fact

About one in 90 births results in twins. If fraternal twins run in your family your chances are slightly higher. Multiple births have increased rapidly, however, due to fertility treatments that involve implanting more than one embryo.

Thoughts and Feelings…

....

....

....

....

....

....

....

....

....

....

DIARY DATES: ....

....

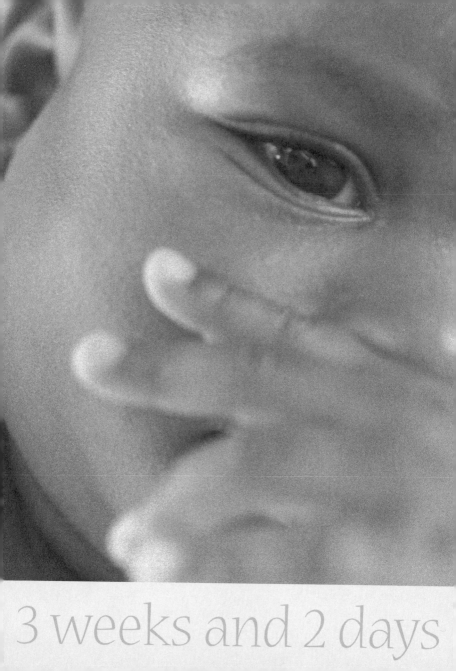

3 weeks and 2 days

day 23

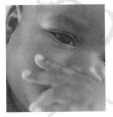

Giving Birth

A fetal monitor in used to measure the baby's heartbeat and the mother's contractions. The monitor, which is usually external, but may also be internal (especially if you are a high-risk pregnancy), indicates how much the contractions are affecting the baby's heartbeat. If it is too much, the delivery is induced with drugs that cause you to deliver quickly, or, in cases of emergency, a Cesarean may be recommended. Internal monitors in particular can restrict movement during labour.

Thoughts and Feelings...

....
....
....
....
....
....
....
....

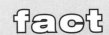

The average fetal heart rate is 120–160 beats per minute (bpm). However, during contractions or other types of stimulation or during sleep cycles, you may get unusual readings of as little as 25 beats per minute.

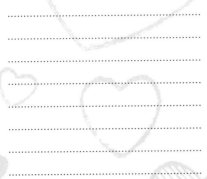

DIARY DATES: ....

....

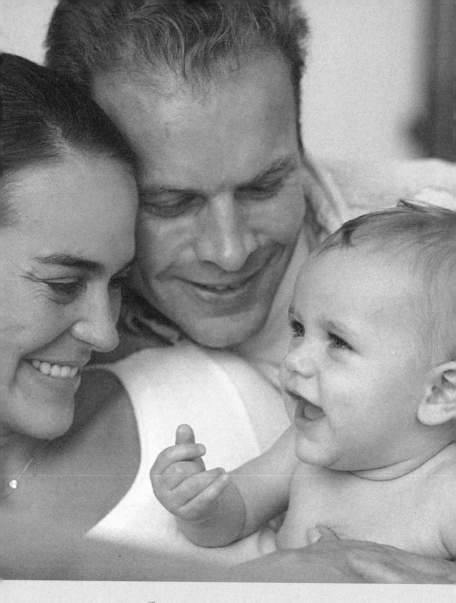

3 weeks and 3 days

day 24

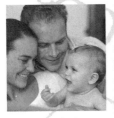

Health and Fitness

Smoking during pregnancy is bad, not only for you, but also for your developing baby. Babies born to smokers (this is either parent!) are more likely to miscarry, be premature, or be of a low birth weight. After birth exposure to smokers can increase the risk of Sudden Infant Death Syndrome (SIDS). Quitting smoking is tough, but now you have the health of your baby as an extra motivation.

Thoughts and Feelings...

....
....
....
....
....
....
....
....
....

WARNING

IF YOU ARE ALREADY PREGNANT AND CONSIDERING QUITTING SMOKING WITH THE HELP OF NICOTINE REPLACEMENT THERAPY (NRT), BE SURE TO TALK TO YOUR DOCTOR. UNDERGOING NRT HAS SIDE EFFECTS FOR THE BABY, BUT IF YOU ARE A HEAVY SMOKER IT MAY BE AN OPTION.

DIARY DATES: ....
....

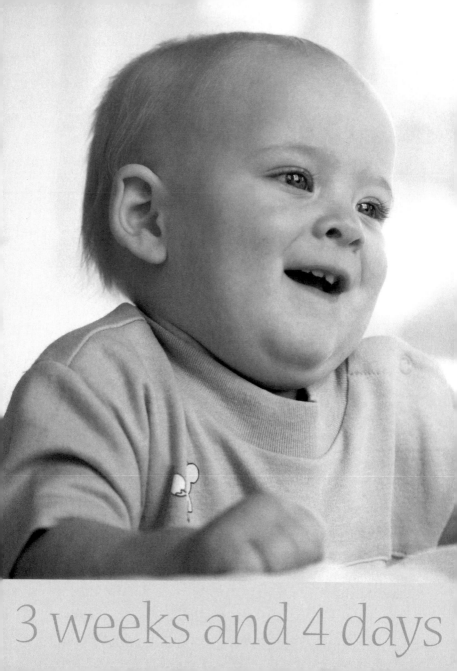

3 weeks and 4 days

day 25

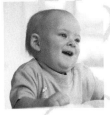

Baby's Development

The blastocyst is made up of two distinct layers. The inner layer of cells will evolve into the embryo, and the outer layer will develop into the placental membrane. About 15 days after fertilization the blastocyst becomes known as the embryo. The embryo is contained in an amniotic sac filled with a warm fluid that the baby floats in until birth. The amniotic fluid also protects the baby from bumps from the outside world.

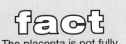

The placenta is not fully formed until the 12th week of pregnancy. Until that time a cluster of blood vessels floats next to the embryo and provides blood at this early stage until the placenta takes over.

Thoughts and Feelings...

....

....

....

....

....

....

....

....

DIARY DATES: ....

....

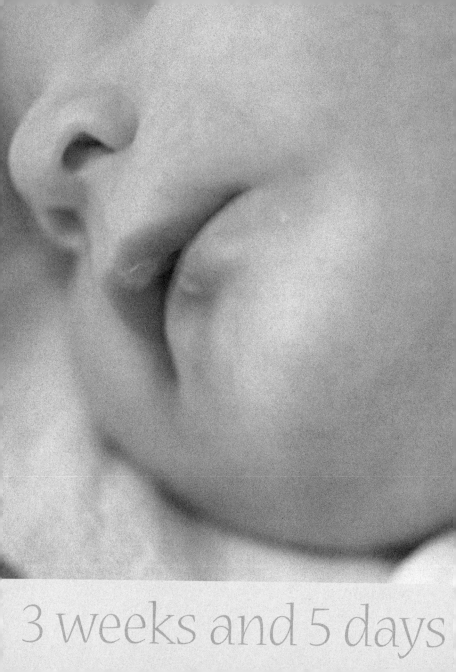

3 weeks and 5 days

day 26

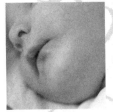

"A mother is not a person to lean on, but a person to make leaning unnecessary."

Dorothy Canfield Fisher

Did You Know?

Your baby's immune system is highly underdeveloped until four months after birth. Breast milk can help to protect against infections. It is also easy to digest—although it cannot rule out colic—and breastfeeding will help you build that all-important bond with your new baby. Benefits for you include a reduced risk of pre-menopausal breast cancer and osteoporosis later in life. In addition, it burns calories and encourages your uterus to shrink—helping you get back in shape more quickly..

Thoughts and feelings...

....
....
....
....
....
....

DIARY DATE: ....
....

tip · tip

COLOSTRUM IS THE YELLOW LIQUID YOUR BREASTS PRODUCE IMMEDIATELY AFTER THE BIRTH. SOME CULTURES HAVE REGARDED IT AS 'DIRTY MILK,' BUT, IN FACT, IT CONTAINS ESSENTIAL NUTRIENTS FOR THE NEWBORN AND HELPS PROTECT THEM FROM GERMS.

3 weeks and 6 days

day 27

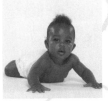

Baby Names for Boys

Barry (Gaelic)
Bartholomew (English)
Basil (English)
Benedict (English)
Benjamin (English)
Bernard (German)

Bill (English)
Bob (English)
Brendan (Irish)
Brett (English)
Brian (Celtic)
Bruce (English)

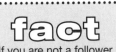

fact

If you are not a follower of a particular religious faith, you may wish to devise your own baby-naming ceremony. You can also ask specific friends and relatives to act as mentors for your child as he or she grows.

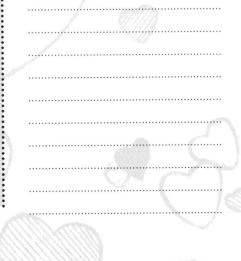

Thoughts and Feelings...

....
....
....
....
....
....
....
....
....
....

DIARY DATES: ....
....

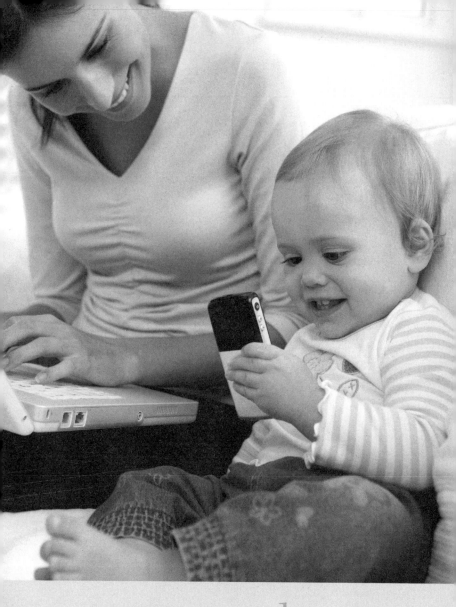

4 weeks

day 28

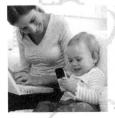

Your Pregnancy

The first sign of a possible pregnancy is when you miss your period. However, periods can be late for many reasons. It is early yet to do a pregnancy test, but, if you just can't wait, some home kits claim to be able to confirm a pregnancy as early as the first day of your next period. Use an early morning sample of urine, as this will contain the highest concentration of the pregnancy hormone, human chorionic gonadotropin (hCG).

Thoughts and Feelings...

....

....

....

....

....

....

....

....

....

Question

How do pregnancy tests work?

Pregnancy tests measure the levels of hCG in your urine. This hormone will not be present until after the embryo is implanted in the endometrial lining of the uterine wall.

DIARY DATES: ....

....

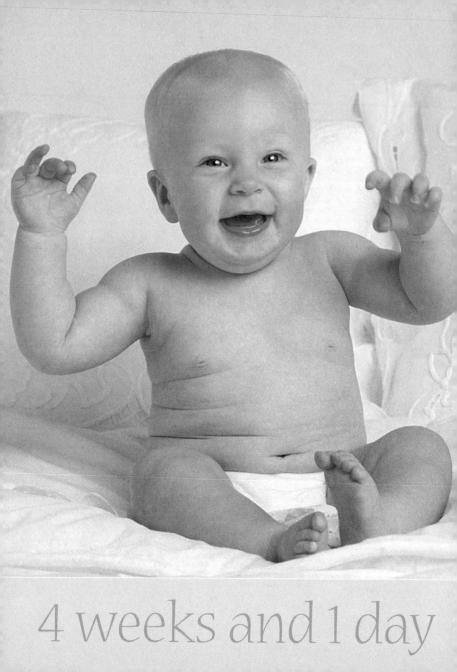

4 weeks and 1 day

day 29

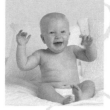

Did You Know?

Identical, or monozygotic, twins come about when a single fertilized egg splits in two. This split will usually happen within days of fertilization, but can happen up to two weeks later. Because they are created from the same genetic material, monozygotic twins will always be the same sex. They may share an amniotic sac and/or the chorionic membrane, or they may have their own space. Fertilized eggs that split after 14 days run a higher risk of becoming conjoined.

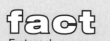

Fraternal, or non-identical, twins created from two separate eggs are three times more common than identical twins. Non-identical twins have their own placentas and are as different as any other two siblings.

Thoughts and Feelings...

....

....

....

....

....

....

....

....

DIARY DATES: ....

....

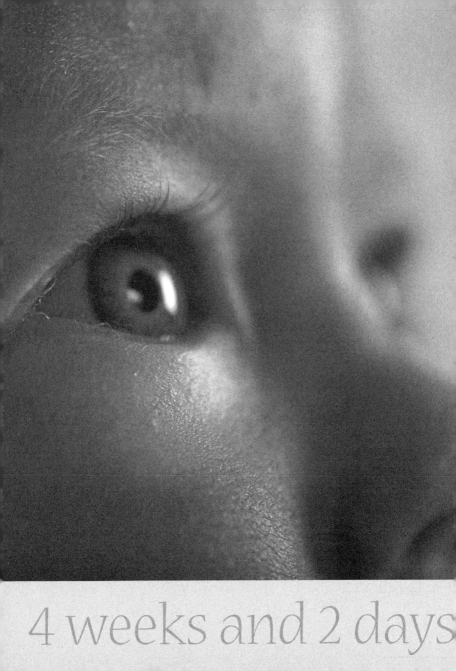

4 weeks and 2 days

day 30

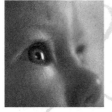

Giving Birth

Nobody knows why a child is born at a specific moment. It may be that the baby relays a signal to the mother's brain as soon as the placenta gives insufficient nutrition and oxygen or if the mother is sick. However, it is not clear why one healthy child is born on time and another stays where it is for a short while longer.

Thoughts and Feelings...

....
....
....
....
....
....
....
....

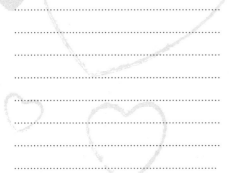

reminder

Past your due date and feeling disappointed that the baby has not arrived? Try to stay busy. If you feel up to it some light exercise, such as a walk, may be just the encouragement the baby needs.

DIARY DATES: ....

....

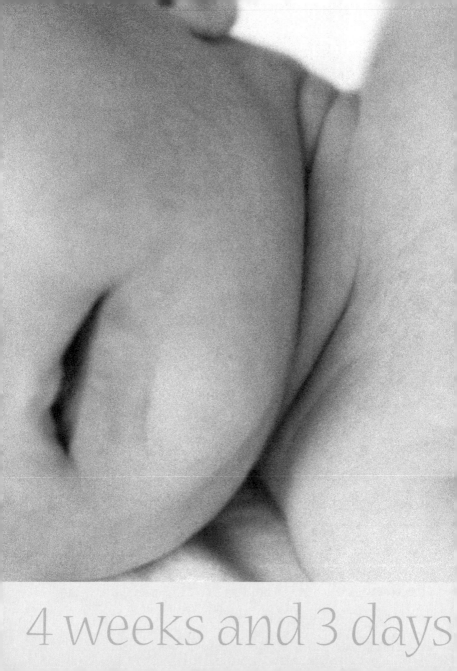
4 weeks and 3 days

day 31

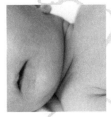

Health and Fitness

X-rays can be damaging to your developing baby. If a doctor or dentist wants to take diagnostic X-rays during your pregnancy, check whether they are actually necessary and ask for a second expert's opinion if necessary. If you work with X-ray machines or CT scanning equipment you will probably need to alter your duties temporarily, and you should be sure to talk to your personnel department about your options.

WARNING

OTHER HAZARDS THAT MAY BE PART OF YOUR JOB BUT COULD BE DAMAGING TO YOUR DEVELOPING BABY INCLUDE HEAVY LIFTING, SMOKY OR EXTREMELY HOT ENVIRONMENTS, CHEMICAL OR IONIZING RADIATION EXPOSURE, AND LONG PERIODS OF STANDING.

Thoughts and Feelings...

....
....
....
....
....
....
....
....

DIARY DATES: ....
....

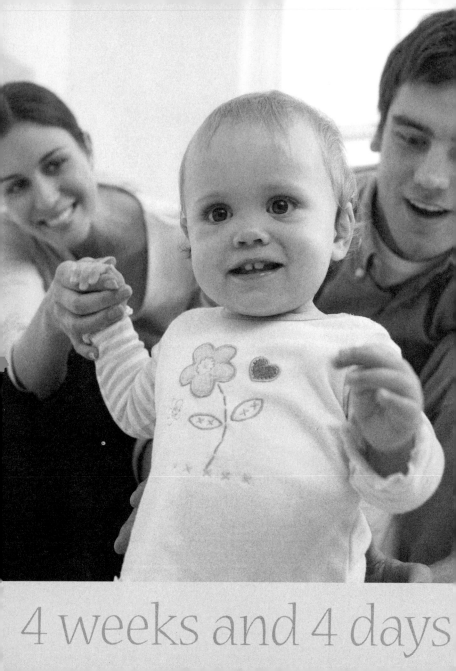

4 weeks and 4 days

day 32

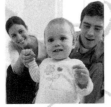

Baby's Development

As the embryo becomes more established in your womb it is secreting more hCG hormone into your system. If a previous pregnancy test was negative, you may now wish to do a repeat test. The embryo is still only $\frac{1}{16}$ in 2mm) in length—and barely visible to the naked eye, but you may already be feeling its impact on your mind and body. Try to get as much rest as you can.

Thoughts and Feelings...

....

....

....

....

....

....

....

....

....

WARNING

IF YOU REGULARLY FEEL FAINT OR DIZZY AND HAVE ABDOMINAL PAIN, CONSULT YOUR DOCTOR IMMEDIATELY, AS YOU COULD HAVE AN ECTOPIC PREGNANCY, A DANGEROUS CONDITION WHERE THE EMBRYO HAS IMPLANTED OUTSIDE THE UTERUS, POSSIBLY IN THE FALLOPIAN TUBES.

DIARY DATES: ....

....

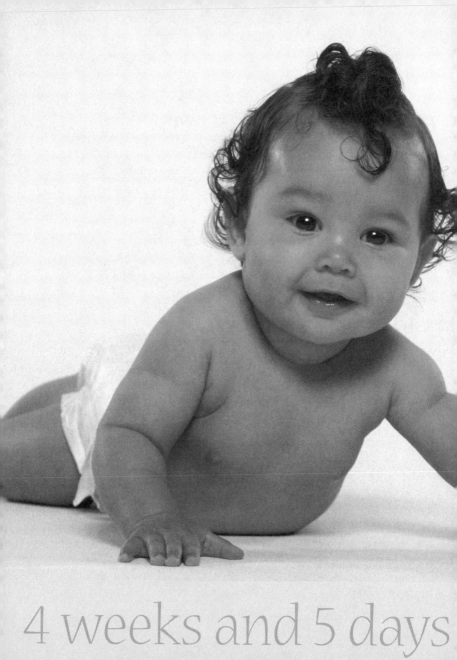

4 weeks and 5 days

day 33

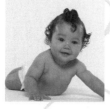

Did You Know?

Dads-to-be are embarking on their own emotional roller coaster as their partner's pregnancy is confirmed. They may feel nervous about the extra responsibility, material and emotional, that is coming their way. Try to share your hopes and fears for the future together. Working together as a family will be the best way to tackle things from now on.

"Fatherhood is pretending the present you love most is soap-on-a-rope."

Bill Cosby, actor and author

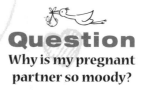

Question

Why is my pregnant partner so moody?

Mood swings in early pregnancy are caused by the many hormonal changes taking place in the pregnant woman's body. If you seem to be being yelled at for no reason, try not to take it personally—the early months, in particular, will be stressful for both of you.

Thoughts and Feelings...

....

....

....

....

....

....

DIARY DATES: ....

....

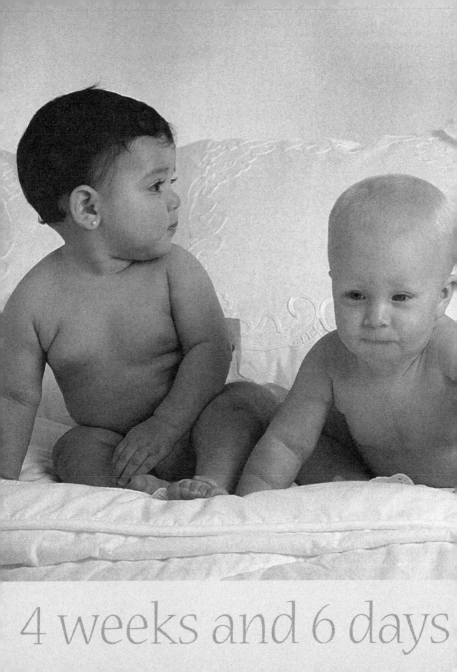

4 weeks and 6 days

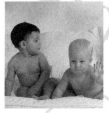

Baby Names for Girls

Carol (German)   Christine (English)
Caroline (German)   Clara (English)
Catherine (English)   Claudia (French)
Chantal (French)   Colette (French)
Cher (French)   Constance (English)
Chloë (Greek)   Courtney (English)

Thoughts and Feelings...

....
....
....
....
....
....
....
....
....
....

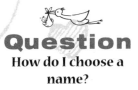

Question
How do I choose a name?

Write down the names you are considering. Make sure you add your last name as well, and then say them out loud to see how they sound. If you are keen on a middle name, add that in as well.

DIARY DATES: ....
....

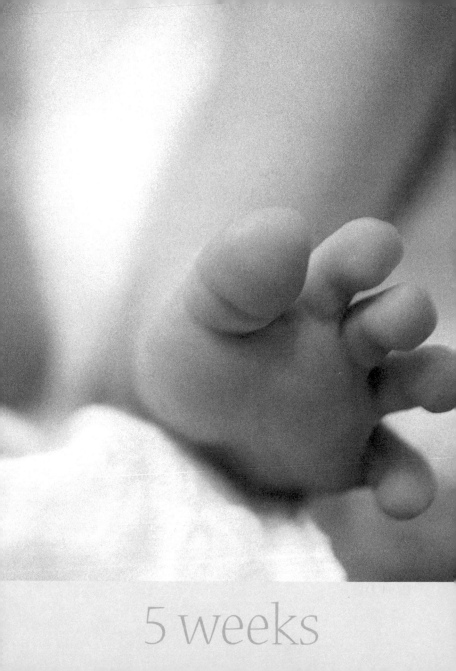

5 weeks

day 35

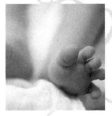

Your Pregnancy

Make an appointment to see your doctor as soon as you know you are pregnant. He or she will confirm the pregnancy, discuss the type of antenatal care available and discuss your options for the birth. A booking-in appointment will be arranged, between the eighth and 12th week of your pregnancy. You may be offered a smear test and tests for sexually transmitted diseases (STDs) and HIV. infection. Take away educational material and study it at your leisure—you will receive a lot of information in the next months.

Question

Why do I have to keep going to the bathroom?

High levels of progesterone relax your bladder muscles in the early stages of pregnancy, leading to frequent urination. Things don't improve, either, because as the baby grows your expanding uterus will put pressure on your bladder.

Thoughts and Feelings...

....
....
....
....
....
....
....
....

DIARY DATES: Doctor's appointment to confirm pregnancy results

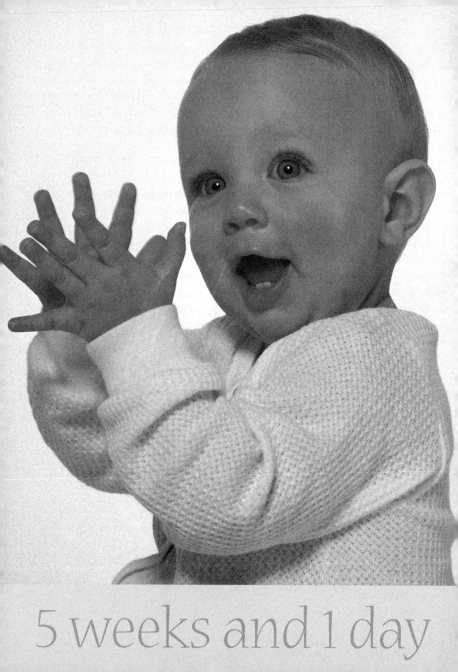

5 weeks and 1 day

day 36

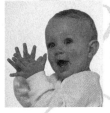

Did You Know?

As the baby grows it will put increasing pressure on your cardiovascular system. Your blood carries oxygen and nutrients crucial to the developing baby, and eventually your vessels will expand to carry an extra 50 percent of blood volume. Your heart will have to pump 30–50 percent more to push this extra volume around your body, and meanwhile your blood pressure will drop. It is not surprising that you may occasionally feel faint.

Thoughts and Feelings...

....

....

....

....

....

....

....

....

WARNING

IF YOU FEEL FAINT, TRY TO REST IMMEDIATELY. SIT DOWN OR LIE ON YOUR SIDE. AVOID LYING ON YOUR BACK, ESPECIALLY AS THE BABY GROWS BECAUSE THE UTERUS WILL PUT PRESSURE ON TWO LARGE BLOOD VESSELS, AND THE RESULT MAY BE THAT YOU FEEL EVEN MORE FAINT!

DIARY DATES: ....

....

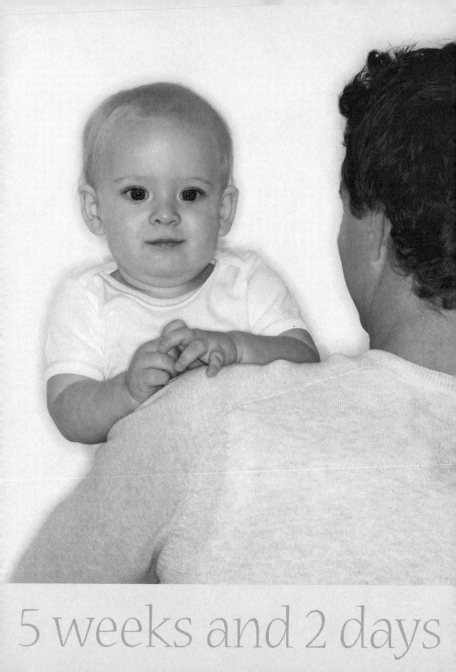

5 weeks and 2 days

day 37

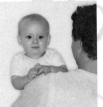

Giving Birth

You may experience 'practice' contractions during the last few weeks of your pregnancy. These are called Braxton Hicks contractions. They actually occur regularly throughout pregnancy, tightening the muscles of the uterus, but you are unlikely to be conscious of them until the third trimester. Unlike real contractions, Braxton Hicks will tend to subside if you change position and move around, and they don't come at regular intervals.

Thoughts and Feelings...

....
....
....
....
....
....
....
....
....

tip · tip ·

MANY WOMEN GO TO HOSPITAL CONVINCED THE BABY WILL ARRIVE AT ANY MOMENT, ONLY TO BE TOLD THEY ARE HARDLY DILATED AT ALL. IT CAN BE VERY DISAPPOINTING TO BE SENT HOME AGAIN, SO TRY TO MANAGE THE EARLY STAGES OF LABOR IN THE PRIVACY OF YOUR OWN HOME.

DIARY DATES: ....
....

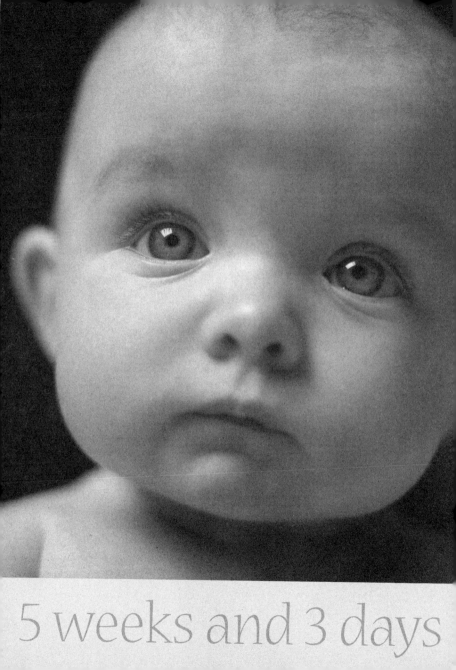

5 weeks and 3 days

day 38

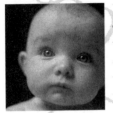

Health and Fitness

Toxoplasmosis is an infection that you can barely notice yourself. You can pick it up through contact with infected cat feces and by eating undercooked meat. You may have built up a natural immunity—especially if you have had pets for a number of years—but if you come in contact with it for the first time while pregnant it can cause brain damage and other problems in your developing baby.

Thoughts and Feelings...

WARNING

CATS ARE REGULAR VISITORS TO GARDENS, SO ALWAYS WEAR GLOVES WHEN GARDENING. IF YOU HAVE A CAT, MAKE SURE SOMEONE ELSE CLEANS OUT THE LITTER BOX. ALWAYS WASH YOUR HANDS THOROUGHLY AFTER BEING OUTSIDE.

....

....

....

....

....

....

....

....

DIARY DATES: ....

....

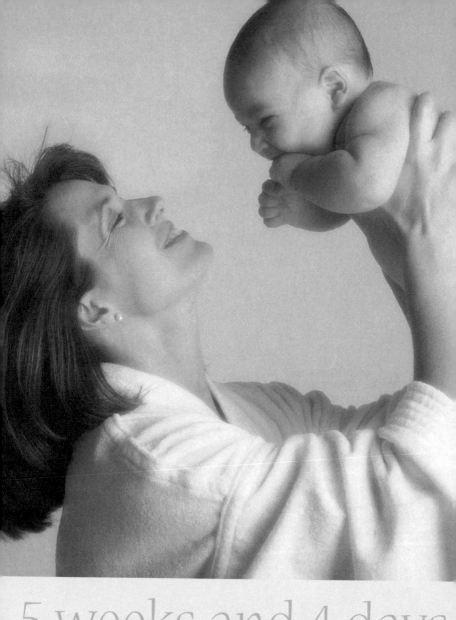

5 weeks and 4 days

day 39

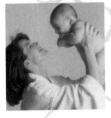

Baby's Development

The embryo now looks like a shrimp. The head, the chest and the belly are forming. Where the eyes and the mouth will be there are small holes. The spinal column and the brain have started to grow. The blood circulation is already working and the heart is beating, although you will not be able to hear it for some weeks yet. The growing baby is just ¼in (6mm) long.

Thoughts and Feelings...

....

....

....

....

....

....

....

....

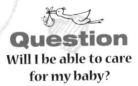

Question

Will I be able to care for my baby?

Even this early in the pregnancy it is common for new mothers-to-be feeling anxious. Try to remember that all new parents learn by experience—although gathering information ahead of time can help prepare you.

DIARY DATES: ....

....

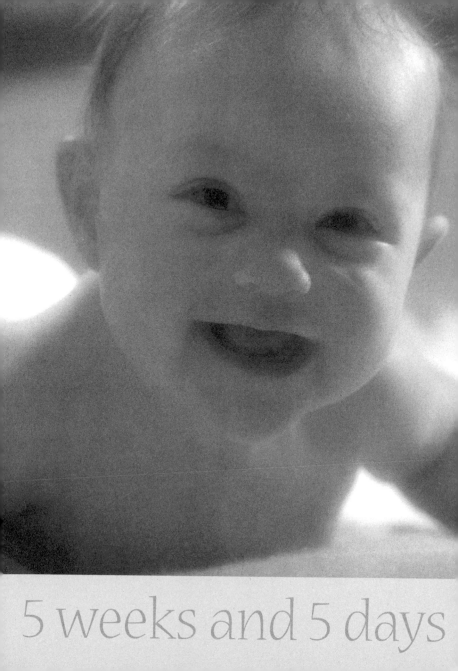

5 weeks and 5 days

day 40

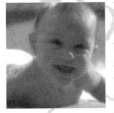

Did You Know?

Until recently, mothers were encouraged to feed and handle their baby according to a strict timetable: crying babies were left to cry for fear of spoiling them. Nowadays we have come to understand that crying is the only way a baby has of communicating its needs, and the mother is naturally programmed to respond to that cry for help. A crying baby may have a dirty diaper, be hungry, or have gas or colic.

"The best way to make children good is to make them happy."

Oscar Wilde, author and playwright (1854–1900)

Thoughts and Feelings...

....

....

....

....

....

....

....

tip · tip · tip · tip · tip · tip · tip · tip · tip · tip · tip · tip · tip · tip · tip · tip · tip · tip ·

IF YOU'VE BEEN THROUGH THE CHECKLIST OF PRACTICAL PROBLEMS THAT MAY BE CAUSING YOUR BABY DISTRESS, IT MAY JUST BE THAT A CUDDLE IS WHAT IS NEEDED. GETTING CLOSE TO MOM IS A HIGH PRIORITY FOR MANY TINY BABIES.

DIARY DATES: ....

....

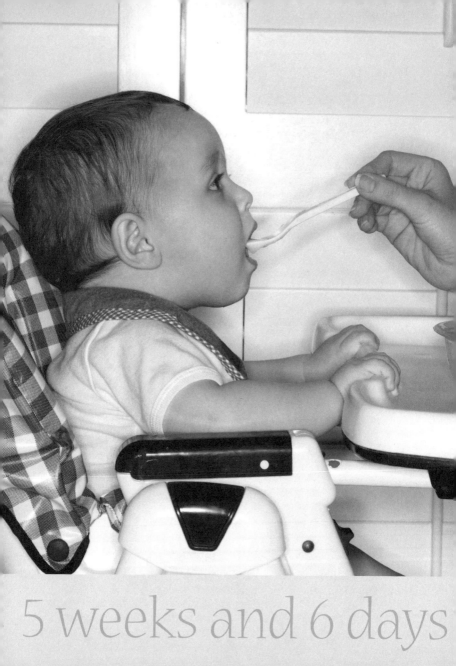
5 weeks and 6 days

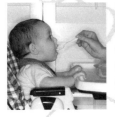

Baby Names for Boys

Cameron (Gaelic)
Cecil (English)
Charles (English)
Christopher (English)
Claude (Latin)

Colin (English)
Connor (Irish)
Craig (Welsh)
Cyril (Greek)

fact

Woody Allen	was born as...	Allen Stewart Konigsberg
Fred Astaire		Frederic Austerlitz
Elton John		Reginald Dwight
Cher		Cherilyn Sarkisian LaPierre
Michael Caine		Maurice Micklewhite

Thoughts and Feelings...

....
....
....
....
....

DIARY DATES: ....
....

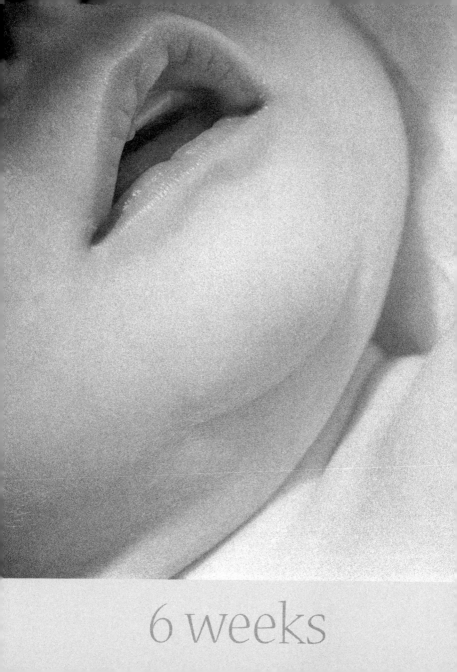

6 weeks

6 weeks

42 days already...

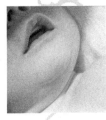

The Mother

Mothers-to-be have a great need for information on everything to do with pregnancy—especially if it is a first pregnancy. There is material available from your care provider, magazines, books and also the Internet. A brief surf around the Web will soon reveal the dizzying number of sites dealing with pregnancy and childbirth. The most effective way to find information is to ask specific questions through a search engine.

Thoughts and Feelings...

....
....
....
....
....
....
....
....

tip · tip ·

USE THE DIARY DATES SPACE TO JOT DOWN IMPORTANT DETAILS, APPOINTMENTS AND INFORMATION AS YOU GO ALONG. YOU MAY FIND YOURSELF GETTING FORGETFUL AND ALSO OVERWHELMED BY THE AMOUNT OF INFORMATION YOU ARE EXPECTED TO TAKE ON BOARD.

DIARY DATES: ....

....

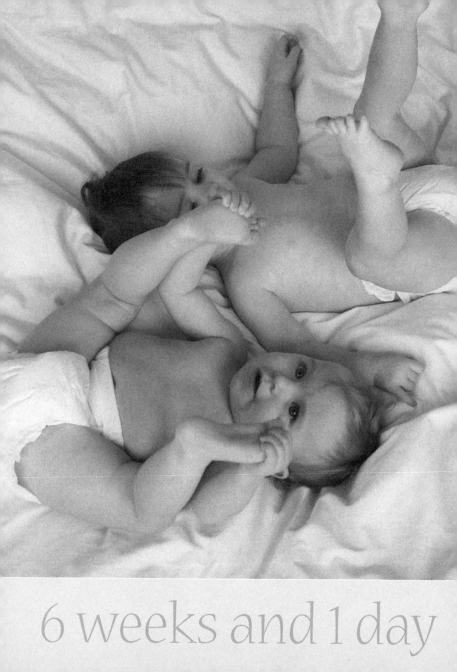

6 weeks and 1 day

day 43

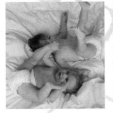

Did You Know?

It can be illegal for your employer to discriminate against you because you are pregnant. (You should check the laws regarding this that apply where you live.) You may be tempted to put off telling your employer until you have passed the 12th week 'just in case.' However, you may miss out on benefits if you put it off. Inform the personnel department or your immediate boss and explain you are telling them in confidence for the time being. You should not be dismissed or treated unfairly at work simply because you are pregnant..

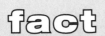

You may be entitled to paid time off for prenatal appointments including prenatal classes, and you should be allowed to take sick leave without its affecting your maternity leave. Be sure to check your company's policies.

Thoughts and Feelings...

....

....

....

....

....

....

....

DIARY DATES: ....

....

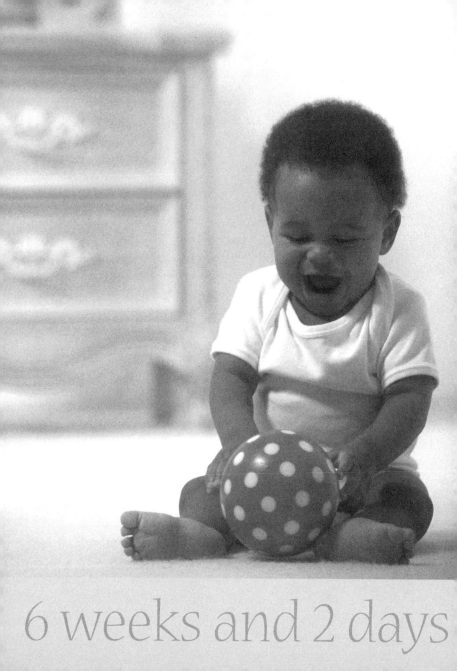

6 weeks and 2 days

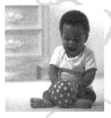

Giving Birth

Because the baby is sitting in a protective sac of amniotic fluid, the pressure of the contractions does not affect him. He does notice that the blood supply becomes reduced, but only begins to experience difficulties when the contractions become longer and more frequent during dilation and later during the pushing phase of the birth. The baby's heart rate may slow down during a contraction but will re-establish itself in the pauses between contractions.

Thoughts and Feelings...

....

....

....

....

....

....

....

....

Question

I have inverted nipples; will this be a problem for breastfeeding?

Nipples come in all shapes and sizes and breastfeeding is always possible. Inverted nipples can be brought out, and large nipples, which may also present a problem, can be worked around.

DIARY DATES: ....

....

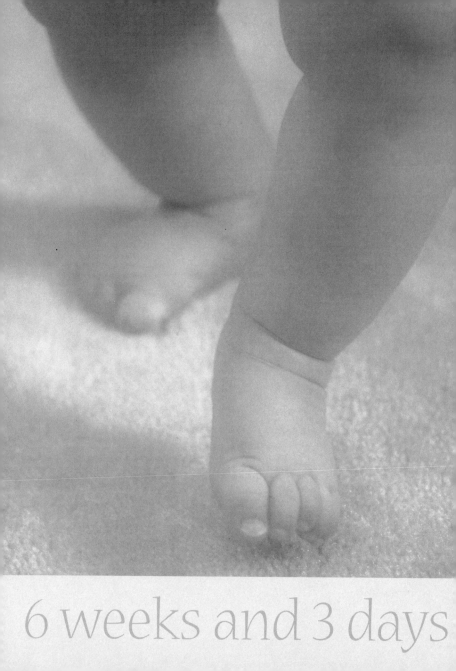

6 weeks and 3 days

day 45

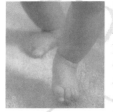

Health and Fitness

Alcohol drunk in large amounts during pregnancy can be harmful to your developing baby. It can cause brain damage and result in low birth weight. Some consider the odd glass of wine during pregnancy to be safe, but you should discuss this with your doctor or midwife before doing so. Many women find that drinking during pregnancy makes them nauseous; this may be nature's way of protecting the baby.

Thoughts and Feelings...

....

....

....

....

....

....

....

....

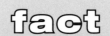

As well as alcohol, you may develop an aversion to tea and coffee during your pregnancy. Strong smells—such as perfume, smoke and fried foods—may also turn your stomach, especially during the first three months.

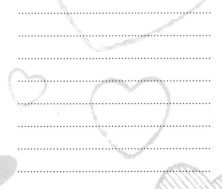

DIARY DATES: ....

....

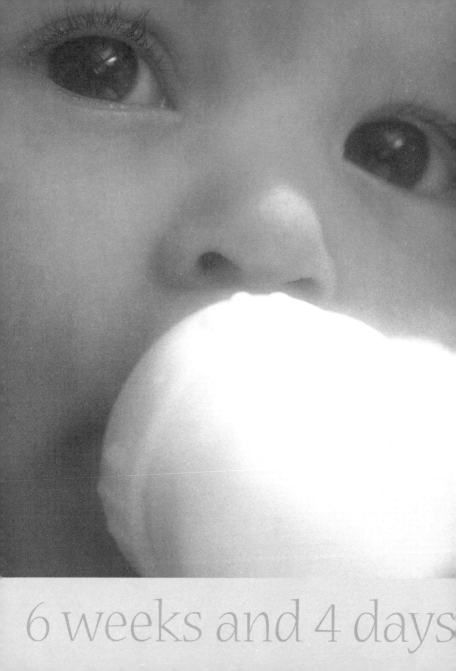

6 weeks and 4 days

day 46

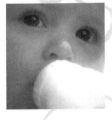

Baby's Development

The fetus is straightening out of the shrimp-like shape it originally was. The intestines are almost completed. The head is changing the most: the ears and eyes are being formed and there are two nostrils and a mouth. The first bone cells are developing and there are tiny buds that will become the arms and legs. The baby is now nearly ¾in (2cm) long.

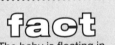

The baby is floating in about ten teaspoons of amniotic fluid. She has plenty of room to flex her growing muscles; however, you will probably have to wait until the second trimester before you feel any of your baby's movements.

Thoughts and Feelings...

....

....

....

....

....

....

....

....

....

DIARY DATES: ....

....

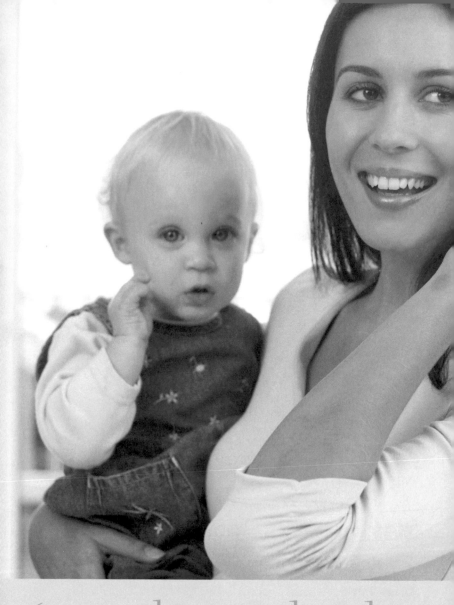

6 weeks and 5 days

day 47

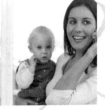

Did You Know?

Changes in skin and hair condition are common during pregnancy. You may develop hair with a shine and a glowing complexion to match, if you are lucky, or you may hit the other end of the spectrum and find you have dull, lifeless hair and skin problems. Hormones are the key to these changes and they are generally beyond your control. Skin pigment can also develop dark patches; to avoid this, use a good-quality sunscreen throughout your pregnancy.

"The only ones who should be allowed to punish their children are those who love them."

Marlene Dietrich, actress and singer (1904–1992)

(taken from *Modern Book of Quotes*)

Thoughts and Feelings...

....

....

....

....

....

DIARY DATES: ....

....

Question

Is it safe to dye my hair during pregnancy?

There is no conclusive proof either way. Some experts recommend not using hair colorings at all during the first trimester. A vegetable-based dye or temporary color may be the safest option until the baby is born.

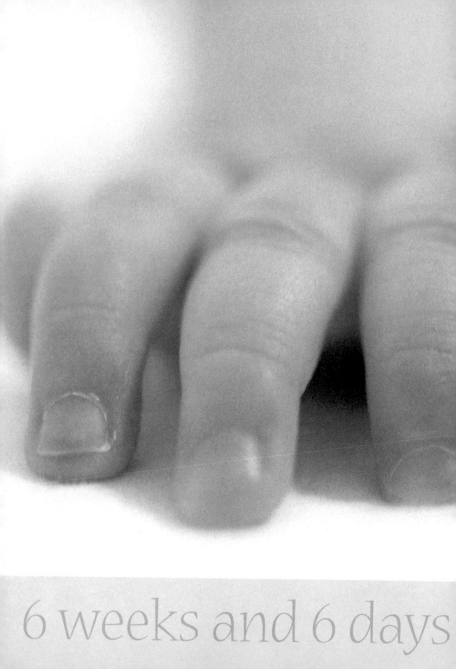

6 weeks and 6 days

day 48

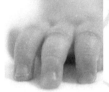

Baby Names for Girls

Daisy (English)
Dana (English)
Danielle (English)
Daphne (Greek)
Dawn (English)
Deborah (Hebrew)

Denise (French)
Diana (Latin)
Dominique (Latin)
Donna (Italian)
Doris (Greek)
Dorothy (Greek)

Thoughts and Feelings...

....
....
....
....
....
....
....
....
....
....

tip · tip · tip · tip · tip · tip · tip · tip · tip · tip · tip · tip · tip · tip · tip · tip · tip · tip

A LOT OF PARENTS WORRY THAT THEIR CHILD'S NAME MAY BE SHORTENED INTO AN UNDESIRED NICKNAME. YOU MIGHT BE WISE TO CHOOSE A SHORT NAME SUCH AS SAM OR BETH IN THIS CASE. BUT TRY NOT TO GET TOO HUNG UP ABOUT IT, AS CHILDREN HAVE A WONDERFUL ABILITY TO SHORTEN THE UNSHORTENABLE.

DIARY DATES: ....
....

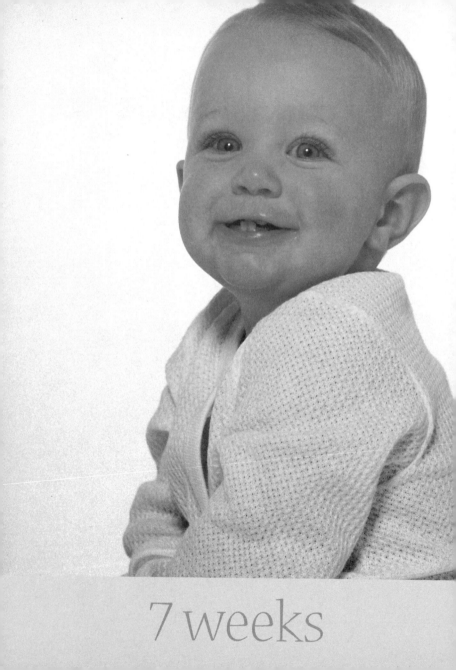

7 weeks

day 49

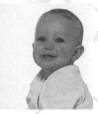

Your Pregnancy

Up to 80 percent of women experience some morning sickness during the first months of pregnancy. Unfortunately, the truth is it can hit at any time of the day—sometimes all day. The good news is, that, for most women the symptoms start to ease between 12 and 16 weeks, although for some unlucky women morning sickness can last throughout the pregnancy. Women carrying multiple births may experience especially intense periods of sickness.

Thoughts and Feelings...

....
....
....
....
....
....
....
....
....

> **reminder**
>
> Eating small, frequent meals can help alleviate morning sickness. And, although healthy eating should be a priority, if you are suffering a lot of vomiting eat food that appeals to you and avoid those that you have a strong aversion to.

DIARY DATES: ....
....

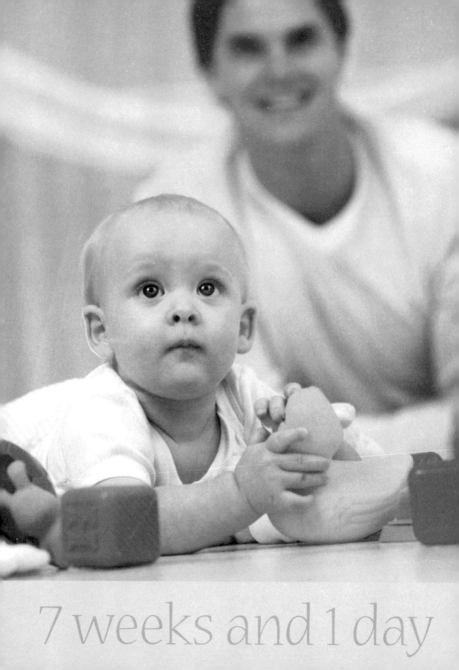
7 weeks and 1 day

day 50

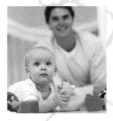

Did You Know?

Many women like to keep a diary during their pregnancy (and maybe even after that, too). After all, in a few years many memories from this special period will be gone: how you picked the name, how friends and family reacted to the pregnancy, how you felt. *Waiting for Baby* provides a format for you to record your thoughts and feelings day by day, creating a diary of treasured memories.

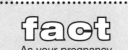

As your pregnancy progresses, you may suffer from forgetfulness. The cause is unclear, but hormones, stress, and sleep deprivation have all been cited. Use the Diary Dates entries in this book to keep lists and a written reminder of appointments.

Thoughts and Feelings...

....

....

....

....

....

....

....

....

....

DIARY DATES: ....

....

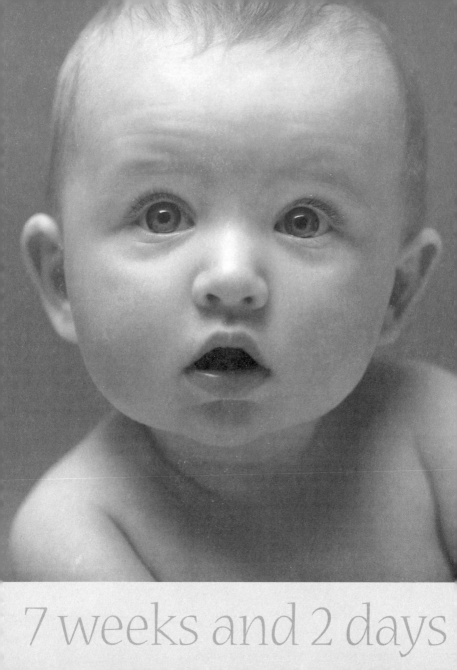

7 weeks and 2 days

day 51

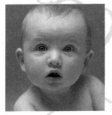

Giving Birth

Once the labor pains start, don't feel you have to stay in bed. Most women feel better if they move around and experiment with different positions. Crawling, kneeling, or squatting can all help or leaning against something or someone and bending forward at the waist. The most uncomfortable position is to lie completely flat on your back; and if you are upright, then gravity will help your baby to descend.

Thoughts and Feelings...

....
....
....
....
....
....
....
....

tip · tip ·

DON'T FEEL GUILTY ABOUT ASKING FOR PAIN RELIEF AT ANY POINT DURING LABOR. YOU CANNOT KNOW IN ADVANCE HOW YOU WILL REACT TO THE PAIN OF CHILDBIRTH—PREPARE YOURSELF BY KNOWING ALL THE OPTIONS OPEN TO YOU AND DISCUSSING THEM WITH YOUR CARE PROVIDER.

DIARY DATES: ....

....

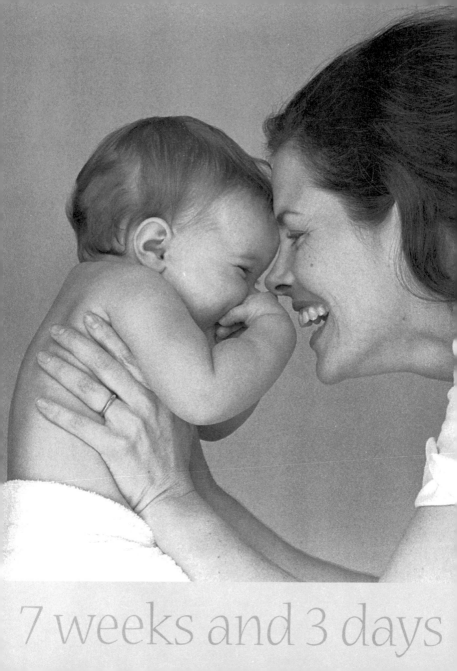

7 weeks and 3 days

day 52

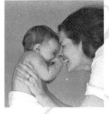

Health and Fitness

Having a baby growing inside you is hard work for your body. At the start of the pregnancy, many woman feel tired and need to sleep, even during the day. Hormonal changes in the body are largely responsible. If you have the opportunity, give in to these urges and rest as much as you can. The need to sleep a lot usually diminishes towards the end of the third month.

Thoughts and Feelings...

....
....
....
....
....
....
....
....
....

reminder

New babies are hard work and are accompanied by sleepless nights. It is best to enter new motherhood in as rested a state as possible. If you can't nap during the day, make sure to make early nights part of your plan throughout pregnancy.

DIARY DATES: ....

....

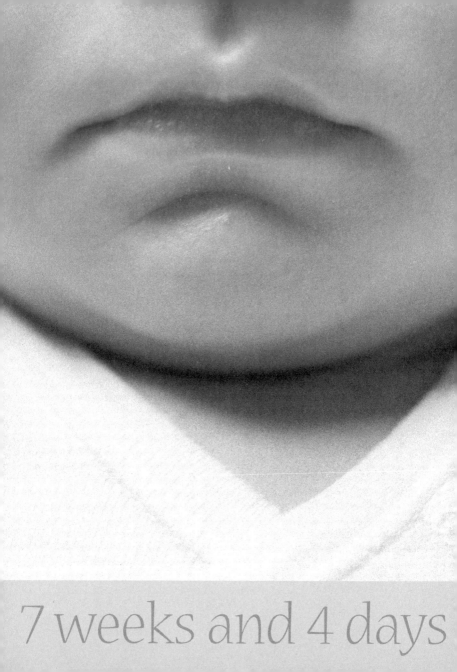

7 weeks and 4 days

day 53

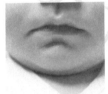

Baby's Development

All the baby's internal organs are in their place. The major joints are identifiable and the spinal column is active; the intestines and brain are almost fully developed, and the brain cell mass is growing rapidly. The lungs are also beginning to develop. Towards the end of the second month the embryonic stage is completed and the baby becomes known as a foetus. It is now nearly 2.5cm (1in) long.

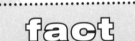

Although the sex organs start to develop around this time, it will not become clear on an ultrasound scan whether you are carrying a boy or a girl until around weeks 16 to 20. Even then, the baby will have to cooperate by lying in a 'revealing' way!

Thoughts and Feelings...

....
....
....
....
....
....
....
....
....

DIARY DATES: ....

....

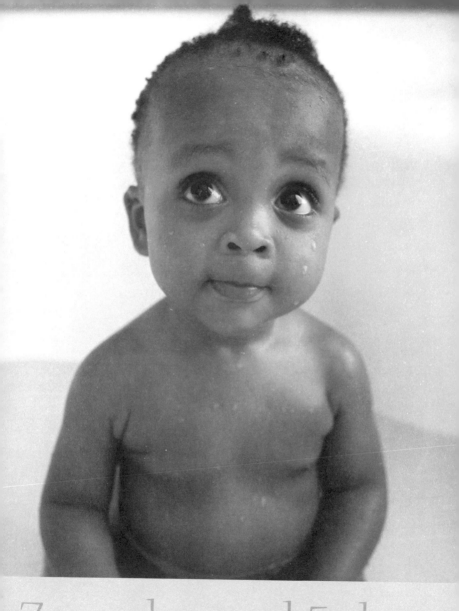

7 weeks and 5 days

day 54

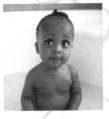

Did You Know?

If you have a toddler already, it may be worth waiting until the first trimester, at least, has passed before letting him or her in on the news of the impending arrival of a sibling. Time passes slowly for very young children. Later in the pregnancy, it may help your first child to prepare for a sibling if you show him or her scans of the baby and let him or her feel the baby move in your tummy.

"When I was born I was so surprised I didn;t talk for a year and a half"

Gracie Allen, actress and comedian (1906–1964)

Thoughts and Feelings...

....

....

....

....

....

....

DIARY DATES: ....

....

tip · tip

IF YOU HAVE ALREADY GIVEN BIRTH, YOU MAY BE IN FOR AN EASIER RIDE THIS TIME. SUBSEQUENT LABORS TEND TO BE SHORTER AND YOU ARE LESS LIKELY TO NEED AN EPISIOTOMY (A SMALL CUT MADE TO ENLARGE THE VAGINA IN ORDER TO AVOID TEARING AS THE BABY'S HEAD APPEARS).

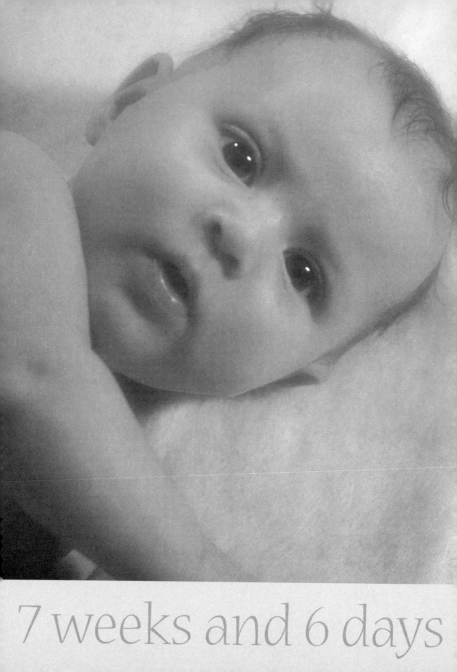

7 weeks and 6 days

day 55

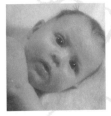

Baby Names for Boys

Dale (English)
Daly (Irish)
Damian (Greek)
Daniel (Hebrew)
Darren (Gaelic)
David (Hebrew)
Declan (Irish)
Dennis (Greek)

Derek (English)
Dermot (Irish)
Desmond (Irish)
Dominick (English)
Donald (Scottish)
Douglas (English)
Duncan (Scottish)
Dustin (English)

Thoughts and Feelings...

....
....
....
....
....
....
....
....
....
....
....

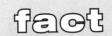

Cultural traditions always play a key role in naming a child. In China, parents sometimes choose what they consider to be a boring or ugly name, hoping that evil spirits will be less tempted to take the baby away into death.

DIARY DATES: ....
....

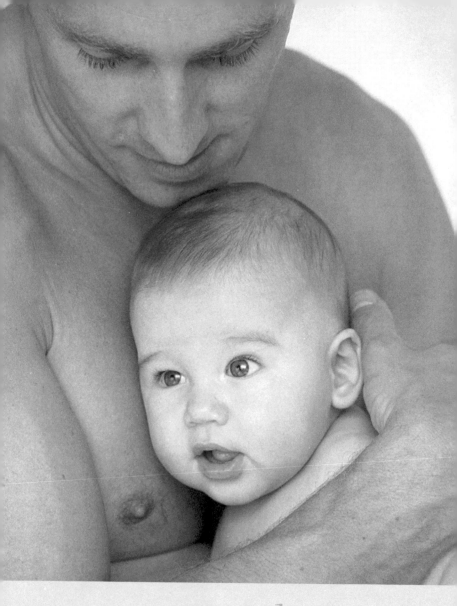

8 weeks

day 56

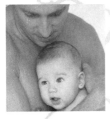

Your Pregnancy

About 20–25 percent of pregnant women lose some blood around the eighth week when your second period would be due to start; this is usually not anything to worry about. Risk of miscarriage is highest in the first trimester and if you have previously had a miscarriage you will naturally be anxious. Make sure your doctor or other care provider are aware of your history and they will follow your progress carefully.

Thoughts and Feelings...

....

....

....

....

....

....

....

....

....

tip · tip ·

IF YOU HAVE HAD A MISCARRIAGE AND ARE FEELING EXTRA ANXIOUS ABOUT THIS PREGNANCY, TRY DESIGNATING CERTAIN AREAS OF THE HOME – SUCH AS THE BEDROOM—AN ANXIETY-FREE ZONE. IT IS HARD TO LET GO OF THIS TYPE OF WORRY, BUT IT WILL DO BOTH YOU AND THE BABY GOOD IF YOU CAN RELAX A BIT.

DIARY DATES: *A second appointment with your care provider between eight and eleven weeks*

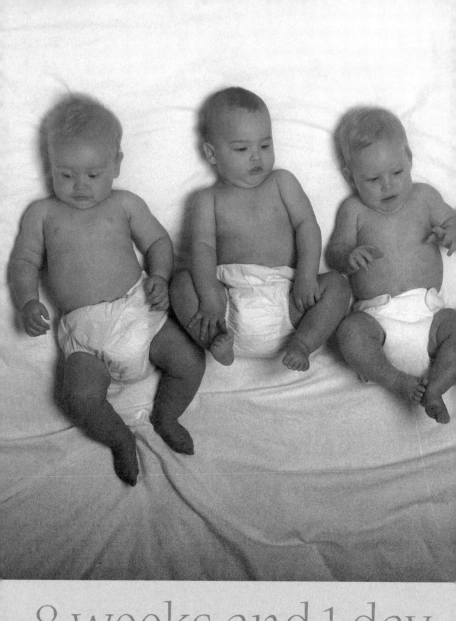

8 weeks and 1 day

day 57

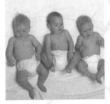

Did You Know?

It is perfectly normal for a pregnant woman to worry about her baby's health from time to time. Still, try to remember that the majority of babies are completely healthy at birth. Four in every 100 babies have a small, non-serious defect and only one in every 100 babies has a defect that is serious.

fact

Your gums will grow thicker and softer due to hormonal changes in your body. Pay special attention to oral hygiene— keeping your mouth fresh will also help if you are suffering from morning sickness.

Thoughts and Feelings...

....

....

....

....

....

....

....

....

....

DIARY DATES: ....

....

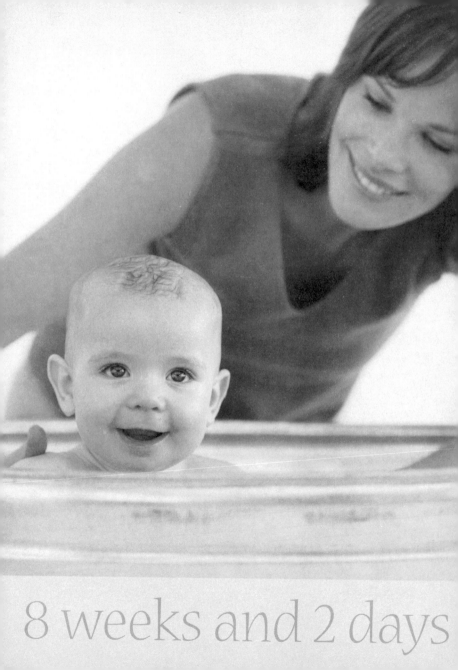

8 weeks and 2 days

day 58

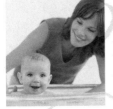

Giving Birth

Nowadays it is the most common thing in the world for your husband or partner to be present at the birth of the baby. Your partner often fulfils a very active role in supporting you both emotionally and physically during labor. However, birth can be a bloody affair and if your partner is squeamish you may wish to arrange for him to leave the room just before the birth.

Thoughts and Feelings...

....

....

....

....

....

....

....

....

....

remember

If the father does not wish to be present at the birth, you can arrange for another birth partner to be with you and support you at this vital time. Any close friend or family member would probably be thrilled to be asked to do this for you.

DIARY DATES: ....

....

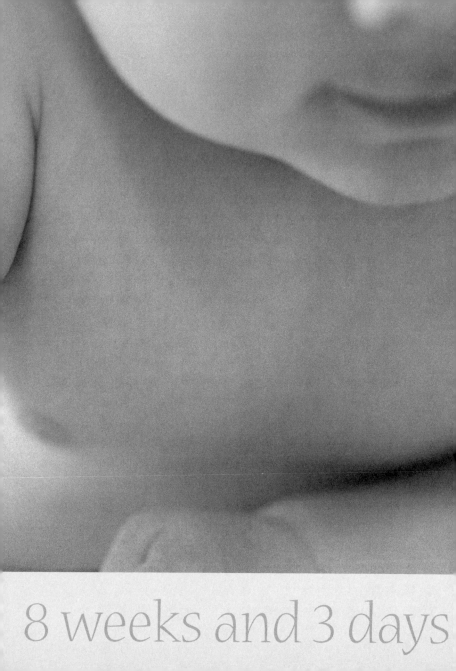

8 weeks and 3 days

day 59

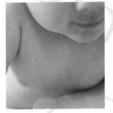

Health and Fitness

If you are suffering from particularly unpleasant morning sickness, there are some remedies that are said to alleviate the symptoms. Ginger is beneficial for nausea so snack on ginger biscuits and herbal teas. Some people swear by acupressure wristbands usually used for travel sickness. Alternatively, it has been suggested that a lack of Vitamin B may lead to morning sickness, so add bananas, rich in Vitamin B, to your diet.

Thoughts and Feelings...

....

....

....

....

....

....

....

....

WARNING

HERBAL REMEDIES HAVE BEEN USED FOR CENTURIES; HOWEVER, SOME ARE KNOWN TO BE DANGEROUS DURING PREGNANCY. ALWAYS CHECK MEDICINES, BOTH TRADITIONAL AND ALTERNATIVE, WITH YOUR CARE PROVIDER.

DIARY DATES: ....

....

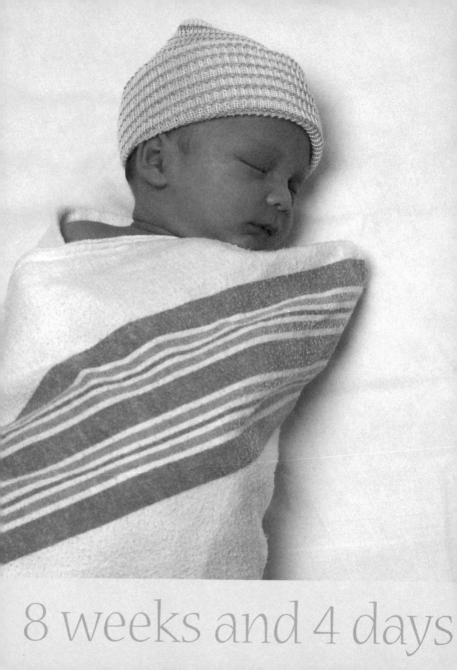

8 weeks and 4 days

day 60

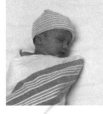

Baby's Development

The limbs are growing fast now, especially the arms. The eventual kidneys are detectable and urine is discharged into the amniotic fluid. You still won't be able to feel it, but the baby is very active now. The face is becoming more defined as it develops and the nose and mouth are clearly visible. The baby is nearly ¹/₁₄in (3cm) long now.

Thoughts and Feelings...

....

....

....

....

....

....

....

....

....

....

reminder

If you are starting to push at the waistline of your clothes you may be thinking about maternity clothes. Remember pregnancy lasts nine months—if you invest in a warm outfit now, it certainly won't see you through to your summer delivery date.

DIARY DATES: ....

....

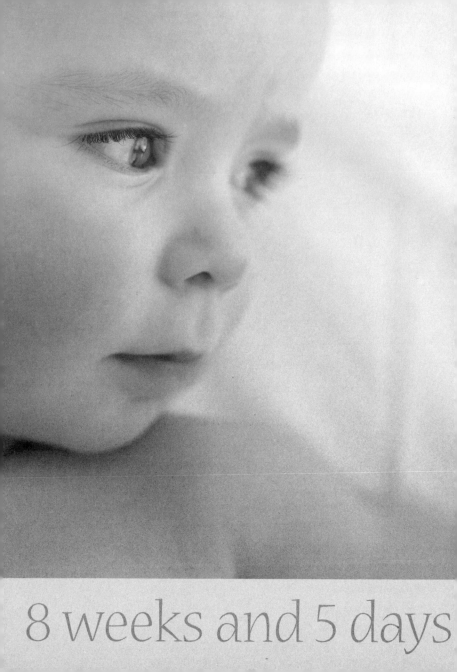

8 weeks and 5 days

day 61

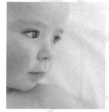

> *"The only sensible way to raise children is by example— admonitory example if necessary."*
>
> **Albert Einstein,**
> physicist (1879–1955)

Did You Know?

The type of care you receive through your pregnancy may depend on the risk category you fall into and what is available in your area. Midwife-led care, with your baby's birth taking place at a birthing center, is available in many areas though not all. When investigating having a birth at a birthing center, look into what additional care will be available (possibly at a nearby hospital) if an emergency situation should arise during the pregnancy or birth,

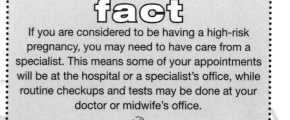

fact

If you are considered to be having a high-risk pregnancy, you may need to have care from a specialist. This means some of your appointments will be at the hospital or a specialist's office, while routine checkups and tests may be done at your doctor or midwife's office.

Thoughts and Feelings...

....

....

....

DIARY DATES: ....

....

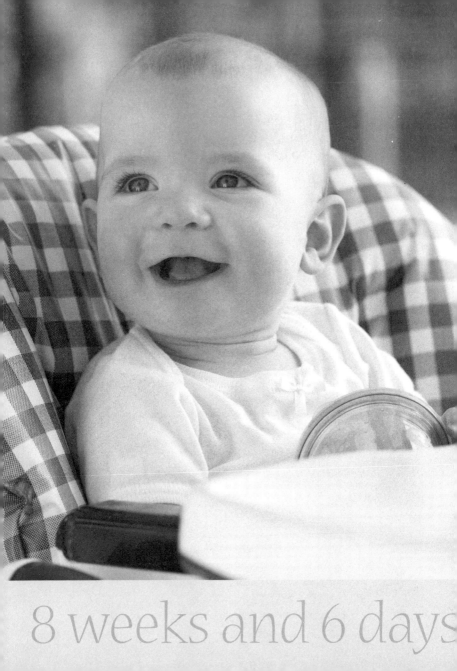

8 weeks and 6 days

Baby Names for Girls

Ebony (African American)
Eden (Hebrew)
Edith (English)
Eileen (Irish)
Ela (Hindu)
Elaine (French)
Eleanor (English)
Elizabeth (Hebrew)
Ellen (English)

Elsa (Spanish)
Emily (English)
Emma (German)
Erica (Scandinavian)
Erin (Gaelic)
Esme (French)
Esther (Hebrew)
Eva (Hebrew)
Evelyn (French)

fact

	was born as...	
Bill Clinton		William Blythe
Elvis Costello		Declan McManus
Bob Dylan		Robert Zimmerman
Alan Alda		Alphonso D'Abruzzo
Billie Holiday		Eleanora Fagan

Thoughts and Feelings...

....

....

....

DIARY DATES: ....

....

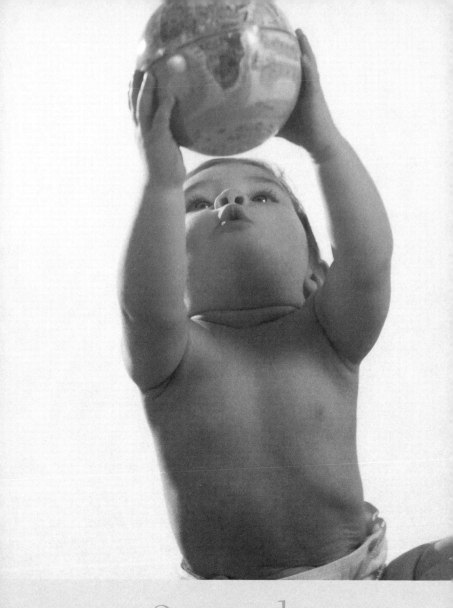

9 weeks

9 weeks

day 63

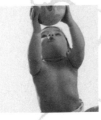

Your Pregnancy

By now, most women can easily tell they are pregnant, both physically and mentally. Physical signs may be nausea, sensitive breasts and extreme fatigue; being weepy and over-sensitive are also typical of this stage of pregnancy. Postnasal drip and/or a stuffy nose plus excessive saliva are symptoms caused by hormonal changes, and they can last throughout your pregnancy.

Thoughts and Feelings...

....
....
....
....
....
....
....
....
....

reminder

Constipation is another unpleasant side effect of pregnancy hormones, which relax the intestines and make them less efficient than usual. To help alleviate the symptoms eat plenty of fiber and fruit and vegetables and drink plenty of water.

DIARY DATES: ....
....

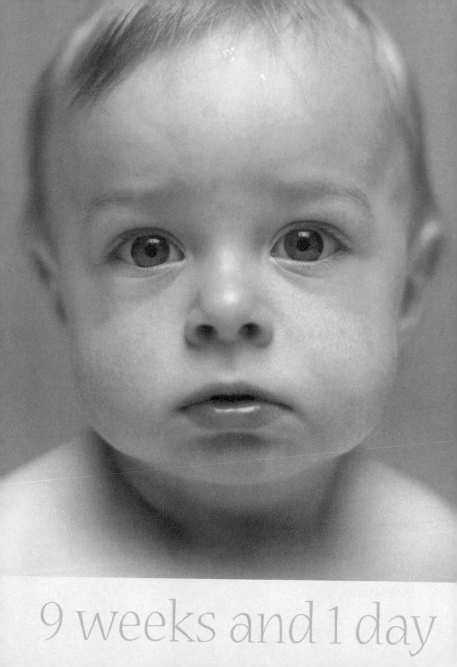

9 weeks and 1 day

day 64

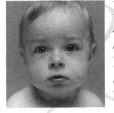

Did You Know?

At your first prenatal appointment you are asked many questions and a full medical history is taken. If you have questions to ask, this is a good time to do so. Make a list before you go, as it is easy to forget when so many things are going on at one time. A blood sample will be taken to identify your blood group, and check if you are immune to rubella (German measles)—which can be a risk to your baby if you contract it during pregnancy.

WARNING

YOUR BLOOD'S RH FACTOR WILL BE CHECKED. IF IT IS NEGATIVE AND YOUR BABY IS POSITIVE, THERE IS A RISK THAT, SHOULD THE BLOODS COMBINE, YOUR IMMUNE SYSTEM WILL REACT AS IF THERE IS AN INTRUDER AND THIS CAN CAUSE SERIOUS COMPLICATIONS. YOUR CARE PROVIDER SHOULD DISCUSS WITH YOU WHAT STEPS MAY NEED TO BE TAKEN IN SUCH A SITUATION.

Thoughts and Feelings...

....
....
....
....
....
....
....
....

DIARY DATES: ....
....

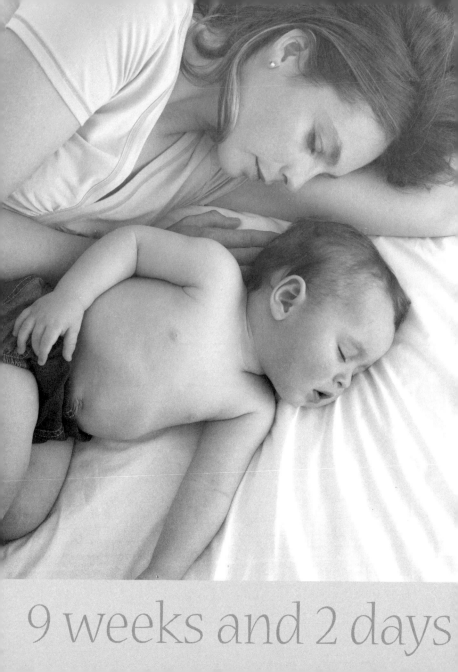

9 weeks and 2 days

9 weeks and 2 days

day 65

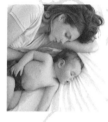

Giving Birth

If you start pushing before your cervix has fully dilated you may already be exhausted by the time your body is really ready to go. In the last stages of dilation the contractions come thick and fast and your body may be giving you a very strong message to push. Take quick shallow breaths and try as hard as you can to resist the urge to push until your care provider gives you the go ahead.

fact

As soon as the baby is born, the womb continues to contract, and since the placenta cannot contract, it automatically becomes detached from the wall of the womb. The entire placenta must be expelled to avoid complications later on.

Thoughts and Feelings...

....
....
....
....
....
....
....
....
....

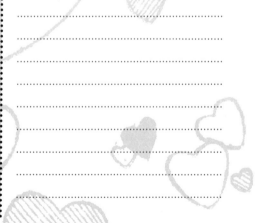

DIARY DATES: ....
....

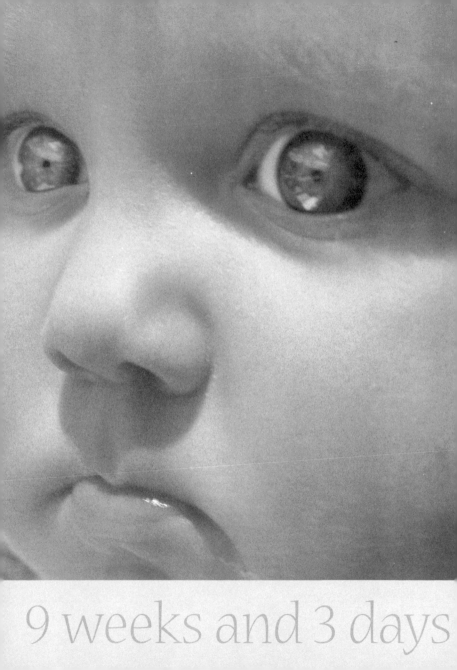

9 weeks and 3 days

day 66

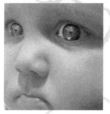

Health and Fitness

Your baby takes all the nourishment it needs to grow from the food you eat, so it is really important to maintain a balanced diet during pregnancy. You need a good combination of starchy carbohydrates (bread, cereals, pasta, rice and potatoes), protein sources (meat, fish, nuts, beans and eggs), and vitamins and minerals from fruit and vegetables. Dairy products such as milk, yogurt and cheese provide essential calcium.

Thoughts and Feelings...

....

....

....

....

....

....

....

....

tip · tip

VEGANS AND VEGETARIANS MAY WANT TO DISCUSS THEIR NEEDS WITH A DIETICIAN. AS THE BABY GROWS AND ABSORBS MORE AND MORE FROM ITS MOTHER IT IS EASY TO BECOMES DEFICIENT IN IRON, CALCIUM, OR VITAMIN B_{12}.

DIARY DATES: ....

....

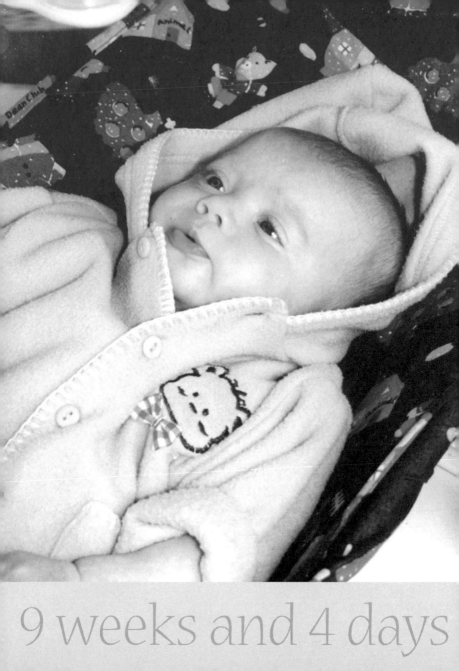

9 weeks and 4 days

day 67

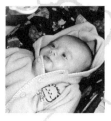

Baby's Development

The head is big in relation to the rest of the body and is growing fast to make room for the brain – which is also developing rapidly. The fingers and toes are identifiable, but still connected to each other by skin. The eyes are almost fully developed and the mouth and nose are showing clearly. The foetus is now nearly 4.5cm (1¾in) long.

Thoughts and Feelings...

....
....
....
....
....
....
....
....
....
....

tip · tip · tip · tip · tip · tip · tip · tip · tip · tip · tip · tip · tip · tip · tip · tip · tip · tip · tip · tip

IF YOU DON'T WANT TO SPEND A FORTUNE ON MATERNITY CLOTHES, USE A LITTLE IMAGINATION. IS THERE ANYTHING IN YOUR PARTNER'S CLOSET THAT YOU COULD BORROW FOR THE DURATION? DO YOU HAVE FRIENDS WHO HAVE RECENTLY BEEN PREGNANT? PERHAPS YOU COULD BORROW OR BUY SOME CLOTHES FROM THEM.

DIARY DATES: ....
....

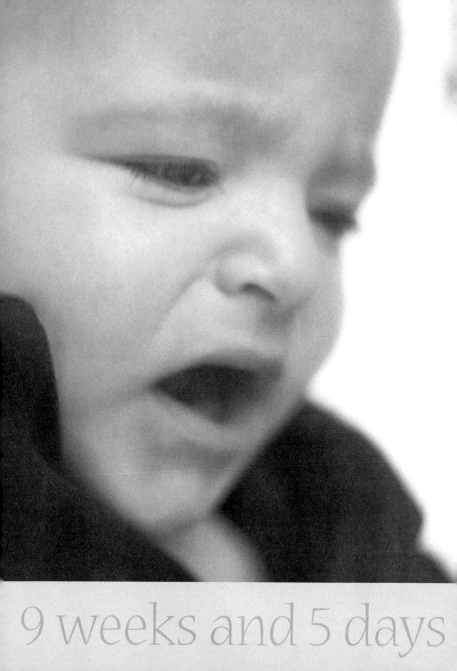

9 weeks and 5 days

day 68

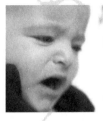

Did You Know?

You may be offered a nuchal translucency test for Down Syndrome. It is carried out at 10–14 weeks and measures, by ultrasound scan, the fold of skin at the back of the neck of the fetus. This measurement is combined with your age and hormone levels in your blood to give a risk factor. More intrusive—but more accurate tests—such as amniocentesis or chorionic villus sampling (CVS) will then be offered.

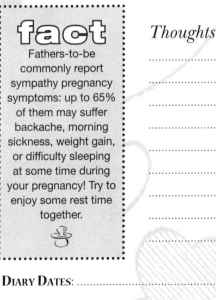

fact

Fathers-to-be commonly report sympathy pregnancy symptoms: up to 65% of them may suffer backache, morning sickness, weight gain, or difficulty sleeping at some time during your pregnancy! Try to enjoy some rest time together.

Thoughts and Feelings...

....

....

....

....

....

....

....

....

....

DIARY DATES: ....

....

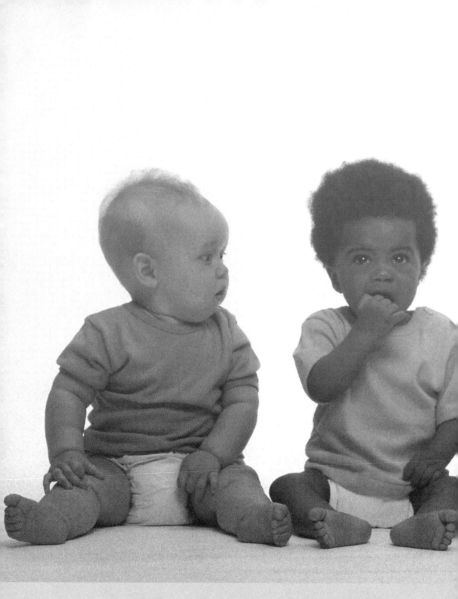

9 weeks and 6 days

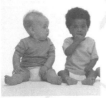

Baby Names for Boys

Earl (English)
Edgar (English)
Edward (English)
Eli (Hebrew)
Elliot (English)
Elmer (English)
Emanuel (Hebrew)
Emerson (German)

Emile (French)
Emlyn (Welsh)
Eric (Scandinavian)
Ernest (English)
Ethan (Hebrew)
Eugene (Greek)
Evan (Welsh)
Ezra (Hebrew)

Thoughts and Feelings...

....
....
....
....
....
....
....
....
....

tip · tip ·

FOR A TOUCH OF
THE EXOTIC, YOU COULD TRY
A TRADITIONAL NAME IN AN
OVERSEAS VERSION: FOR EXAMPLE, PAUL
BECOMES PAVEL IN POLISH.

DIARY DATES: ....

....

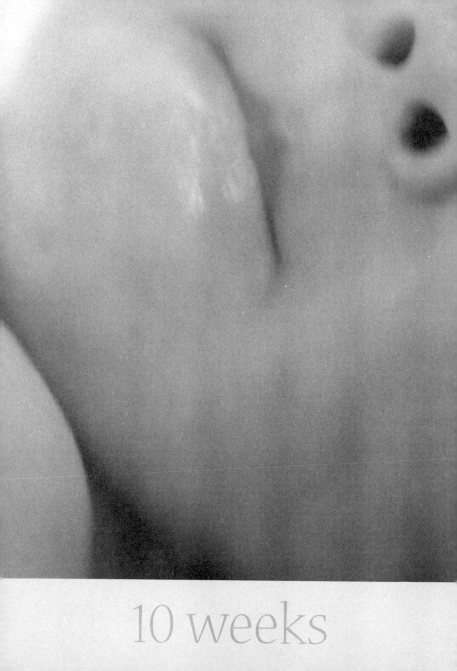

10 weeks

day 70

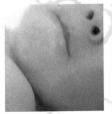

Your Pregnancy

Wearing a seatbelt is compulsory, even during pregnancy. Many women have the idea that wearing a seatbelt is bad for the baby because the belt presses on the stomach. This is not true. The lap belt should be positioned under your bump and the shoulder belt falls between your breasts. It is much more dangerous, for you and the baby, to risk being thrown into the dashboard or through the windshield if you travel without a seatbelt.

WARNING

BABY AND CHILD CAR SEATS ARE COMPULSORY. YOUR BABY MUST RIDE IN A REAR-FACING CAR SEAT UNTIL HE WEIGHS AT LEAST 20LB (9KG). DON'T BUY SECOND-HAND CAR SEATS—YOU DON'T KNOW IF THEY HAVE BEEN IN AN ACCIDENT AND IT IS NOT ALWAYS POSSIBLE TO TELL IF THEY HAVE BEEN DANGEROUSLY DAMAGED.

Thoughts and Feelings...

....

....

....

....

....

....

....

....

DIARY DATES: ....

....

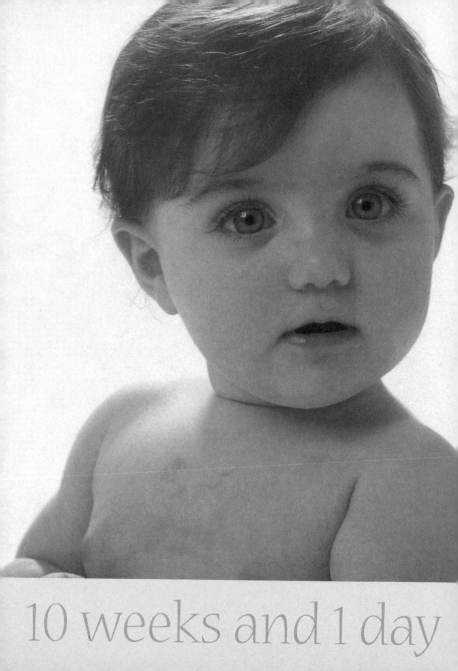

10 weeks and 1 day

day 71

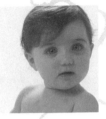

Did You Know?

Your blood pressure and a urine sample will be tested at every antenatal check-up. An elevated blood pressure can indicate pre-eclampsia, which is a dangerous condition for both you and the baby. Urine is checked for infections that may need treatment. Protein may again indicate pre-eclampsia. Sugar could be a sign of diabetes and ketones may indicate that your liver is struggling to cope with your pregnancy.

Thoughts and Feelings...

....

....

....

....

....

....

....

....

....

reminder

You may be given a maternity record file at your first prenatal visit. (If not, then start a file yourself with copies of all relevant records and information.) Such a file will record your medical history throughout the pregnancy. Keep it with you at all times, then if you are away from home your history and a record of the tests you have had are readily available.

DIARY DATES: ....

....

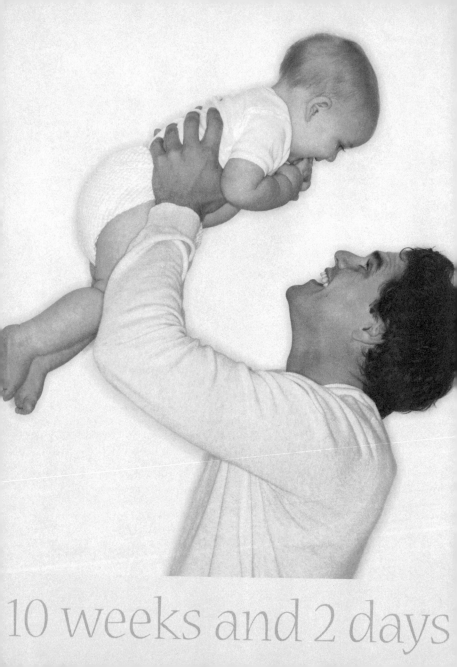

10 weeks and 2 days

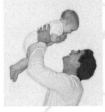

Giving Birth

You may choose to employ a doula to help you through your pregnancy, labor and birth. This is a qualified and experienced woman who will help you make choices on the type of care and delivery you want and act as an intermediary between you and medical staff, which may be a relief to your partner who might otherwise have to do it. She can also help you establish a breastfeeding regimen after the birth.

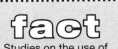

Studies on the use of doulas have shown that they contribute to a reduction in the time of labor as well as significantly reducing the amount of medical intervention that can occur during birth.

Thoughts and Feelings...

....

....

....

....

....

....

....

....

DIARY DATES: ....

....

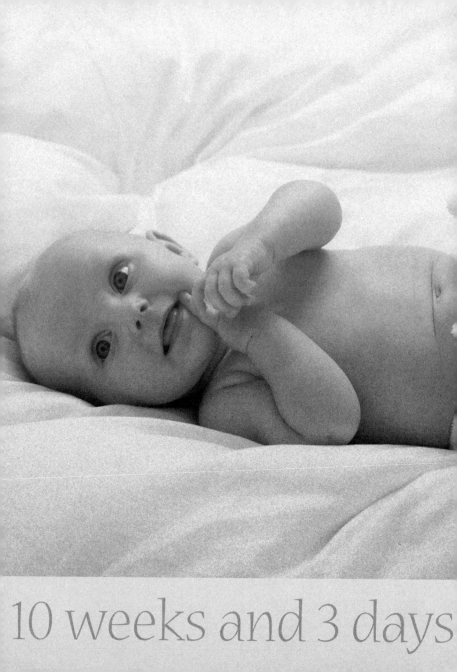

10 weeks and 3 days

day 73

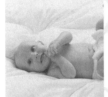

Health and Fitness

Haemorrhoids, also known as piles, can be another side effect of pregnancy. They are a form of varicose vein – which may also occur in the legs during pregnancy – resulting in blocked rectal veins which may become itchy and painful, perhaps even protruding from the anus. Stick to the high fibre diet and drink plenty of water to avoid straining when going to the toilet. They should resolve themselves a few weeks after pregnancy: if they don't, be sure to talk to your doctor.

Thoughts and Feelings...

....

....

....

....

....

....

....

....

tip · tip ·

AN ICE PACK WRAPPED IN A TOWEL OR A WITCH HAZEL COMPRESS APPLIED TO PILES MAY HELP RELIEVE THE PAIN. THERE ARE ALSO OVER-THE-COUNTER CREAMS AVAILABLE, BUT REMEMBER TO CHECK WITH YOUR DOCTOR FIRST.

DIARY DATES: ....

....

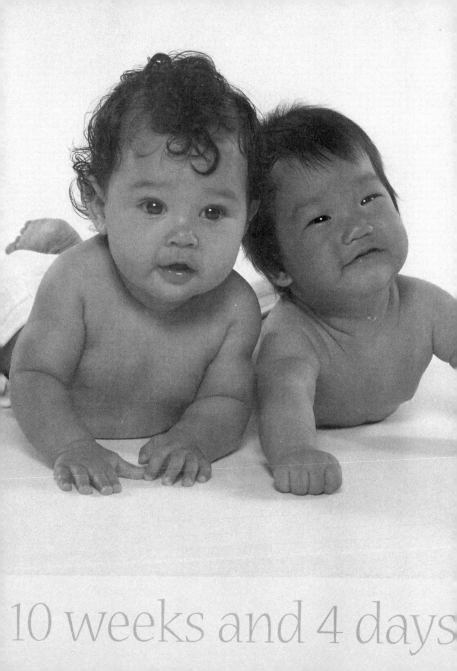

10 weeks and 4 days

day 74

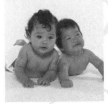

Baby's Development

Although they are still not detectable on the ultrasound scan, the ovaries and testicles are now being created, as well as the external genitalia. However, with the ultrasound scan you can now listen to the heartbeat of the fetus. The chance of damage due to infections, chemical substances, or drugs is reduced now, although rubella (German measles) is still a risk. The fetus is around 2⅛in (5.5cm) long.

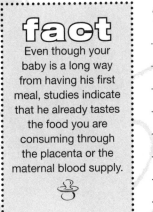

fact

Even though your baby is a long way from having his first meal, studies indicate that he already tastes the food you are consuming through the placenta or the maternal blood supply.

Thoughts and Feelings...

....
....
....
....
....
....
....
....

DIARY DATES: ....
....

10 weeks and 5 days

day 75

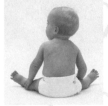

Did You Know?

Trying to look your best may improve your self-image at a time when you could be feeling vulnerable on the looks front. This doesn't mean struggling into the latest fashion statement, but it could mean investing in stylish but truly comfortable sweatpants or a cool dress if you are having a summer pregnancy. If your skin pigment is being affected by pregnancy a good foundation may help even your skin tone.

Thoughts and Feelings…

....

....

....

....

....

....

....

....

....

"I'm open to the idea of having a relationship and starting a family. Someone once told me that the best preparation for motherhood is being a mother to yourself. Just learn to look after yourself first."

Geri Halliwell, singer (taken from *Cosmopolitan*)

DIARY DATES: ....

....

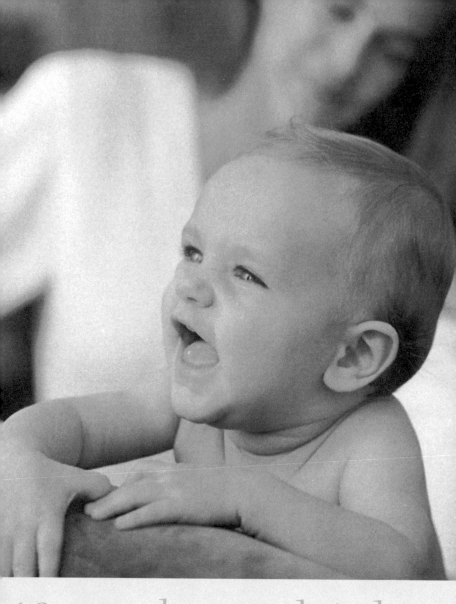

10 weeks and 6 days

76 days already...

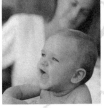

Baby Names for Girls

Faith (English)
Fatima (Arabic)
Fay (French)
Felicia (Latin)
Finola (Irish)
Fiona (Irish)

Flavia (Latin)
Flora (English)
Fontaine (French)
Frances (English)
Freda (German)
Freya (Scandinavian)

Thoughts and Feelings...

....
....
....
....
....
....
....
....
....
....

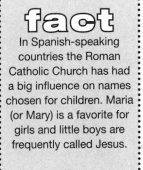

fact

In Spanish-speaking countries the Roman Catholic Church has had a big influence on names chosen for children. Maria (or Mary) is a favorite for girls and little boys are frequently called Jesus.

DIARY DATES: ....

....

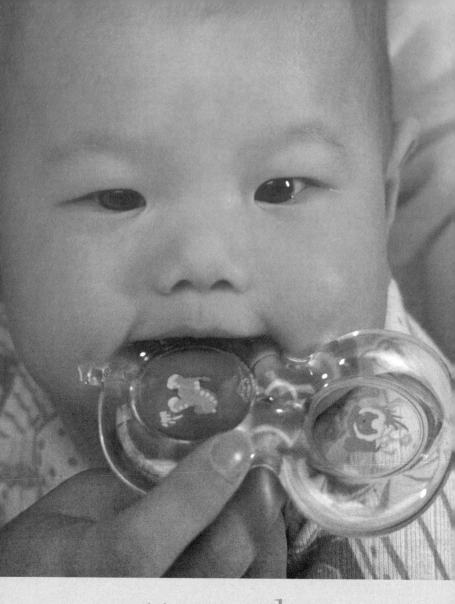

11 weeks

day 77

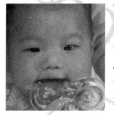

Your Pregnancy

Many pregnant women notice a change in their sexual needs, and this could be either an increase or a decrease. If you suffer unpleasant morning sickness you may not feel too sexy, although this could change as the pregnancy proceeds. Your partner's libido could also be affected. He may be viewing your body as a baby carrier—on the other hand, he may find your expanding waistline particularly sensual. Remember to talk to each other about your changing feelings.

Some couples have a fear that sexual intercourse can harm their growing baby. In a risk-free pregnancy, this simply isn't the case. However, if you have a history of miscarriage or other complications, your doctor may advise you to abstain from intercourse.

Thoughts and Feelings...

....
....
....
....
....
....
....
....

Diary Dates: ....

....

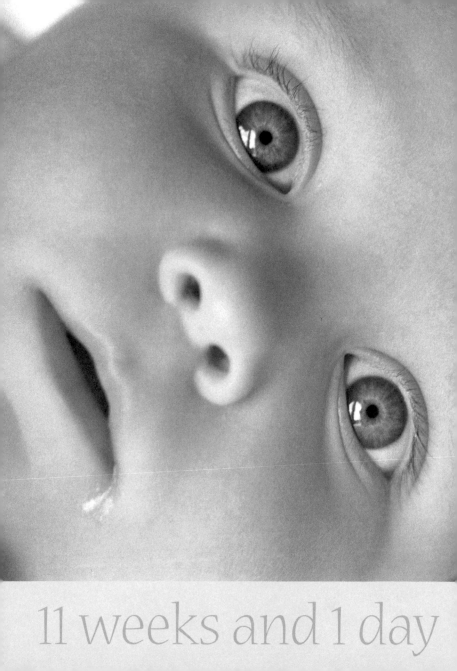

11 weeks and 1 day

day 78

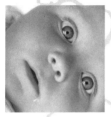

Did You Know?

Your height may be measured at your first prenatal visit, as this can give an indication of pelvis size. Women with a very small pelvis may be advised to have a Cesarean delivery; most babies, however, are in proportion to the size of their mother. Some care providers will check your weight throughout your pregnancy, as a sudden jump in weight can indicate pre-eclampsia.

Thoughts and Feelings...

....

....

....

....

....

....

....

....

....

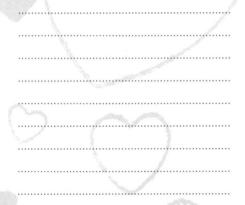

fact

At each prenatal visit, your care provider will check the size of the foetus by pressing your abdomen to find the top of the uterus then feeling down towards the pelvis. They will also be able to tell the way the baby is lying.

DIARY DATES: ....

....

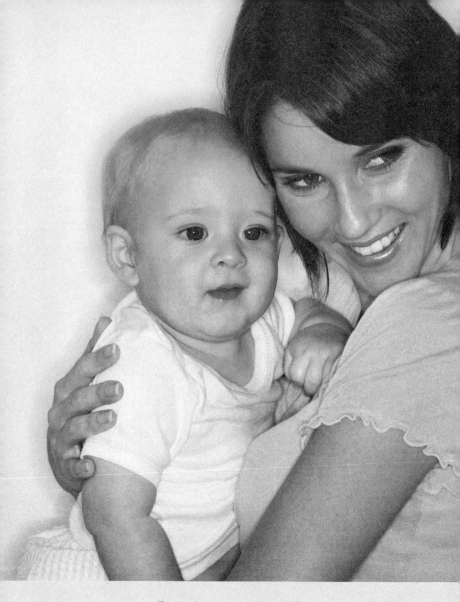

11 weeks and 2 days

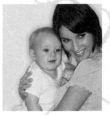

Giving Birth

In most countries, it is standard practice to give birth in hospital, often with the aid of painkillers such as an epidural. in the Netherlands, however, many women give birth at home, and without painkillers. Dutch women can request a hospital birth, or may be advised to have one on medical grounds, but a home birth is accepted as the norm rather than the exception.

Thoughts and Feelings...

....

....

....

....

....

....

....

....

....

....

reminder

Your newborn baby is born with a sucking reflex that can be satisfied by putting him to your breast immediately. The baby nuzzling your nipples will cause your uterus to contract and help to separate the placenta.

DIARY DATES: ....

....

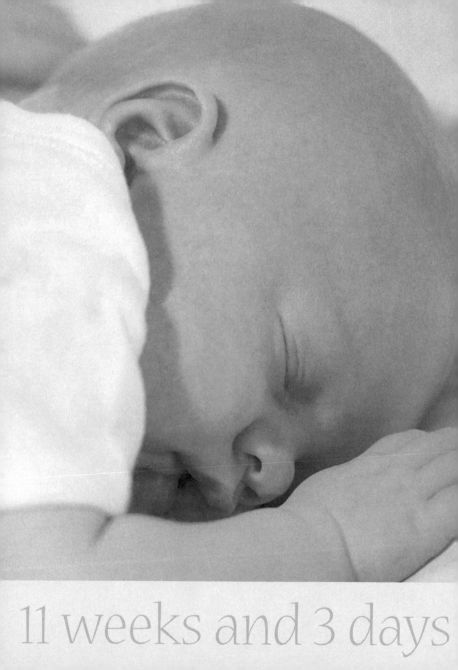

11 weeks and 3 days

day 80

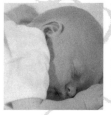

Health and Fitness

Calcium is necessary for the formation of your baby's bone system and teeth. Both during pregnancy and when you are breastfeeding you need extra calcium to fulfil your own needs and those of your child as well. Milk and dairy products are rich in calcium: four 8fl oz (250ml) glasses of milk daily will provide the recommended levels of calcium.

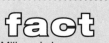

Milk and cheese are the natural choice for your increased calcium intake, however other good sources of calcium are yogurt, broccoli, kale, salmon, almonds, prunes and seaweed. A fruit smoothie is an easy way to boost calcium intake if you are not keen on milk.

Thoughts and Feelings...

....

....

....

....

....

....

....

....

....

DIARY DATES: ....

....

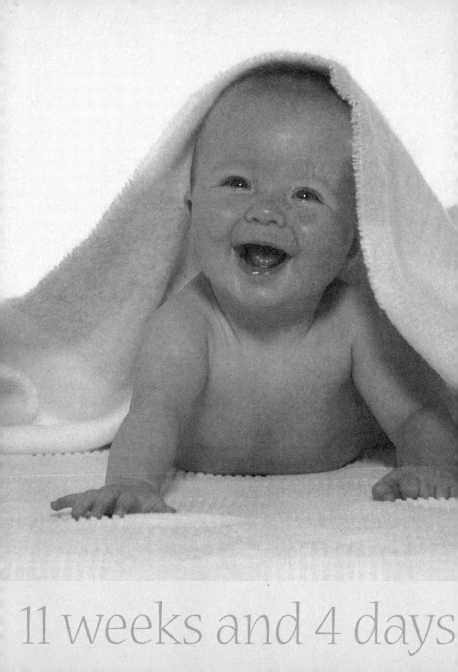

11 weeks and 4 days

day 81

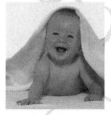

Baby's development

The joints are functioning, the toes are bending and the baby is sucking, and may be sucking its thumb even at this early stage. The fingers and toes already have nails. The baby can swallow and drinks amniotic fluid and passes it back as urine. The baby is now about 2½in (6.5cm) in length and weighs about ¾oz (20g).

Thoughts and Feelings...

....

....

....

....

....

....

....

....

....

....

fact

Your baby is now being entirely nourished by the fully formed placenta (which looks something like a pizza!). The baby is attached to the placenta by the umbilical cord, which feeds it nutrients and oxygen and carries away the waste.

DIARY DATES: ....

....

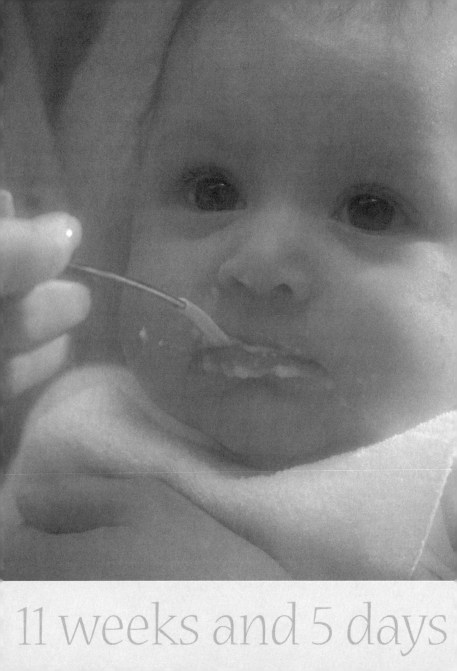

11 weeks and 5 days

11 weeks and 5 days
day 82

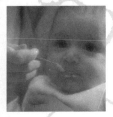

Did You Know?
Writing a birth plan gives you and your partner the opportunity to discuss and decide in detail how you would like the birth to take place. On the day, when emotions are running high and events can become rather frantic, it will help you remain clear about how you want things to proceed. Be realistic, though: anything can happen and things can turn out differently from how you hoped.

"Come mothers and fathers throughout the land, and don't criticize what you can't understand."

Bob Dylan, singer and songwriter

(taken from *Prisma Quotes*)

Thoughts and Feelings...

tip·tip·tip·tip·tip·tip·tip·tip·tip·tip·tip·tip·tip·tip·tip·tip·tip·tip·tip·tip·tip·tip·tip·tip

GO THROUGH YOUR BIRTH PLAN WITH YOUR CARE PROVIDER THEN ASK FOR A COPY OF THE PLAN TO BE ATTACHED TO YOUR CHART AND HOSPITAL RECORD.

....

....

....

....

....

DIARY DATES: ....

....

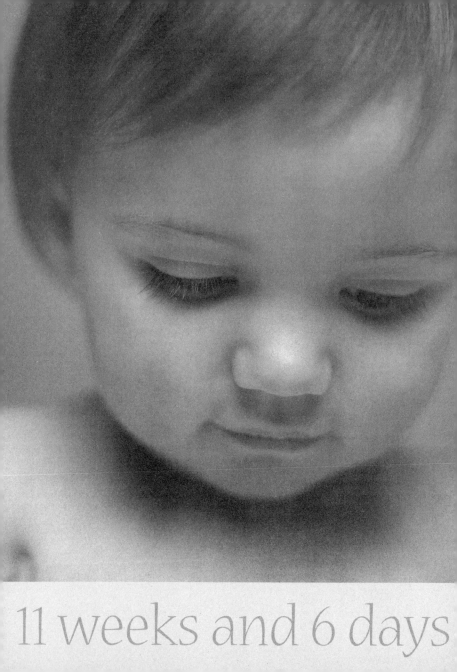

11 weeks and 6 days

day 83

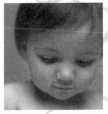

Baby Names for Boys

Fabian (Latin)
Fairfax (English)
Ferdinand (German)
Fergal (Irish)
Fingall (Scottish)
Finlay (Irish)
Finnegan (Irish)

Fitz (English)
Floyd (Welsh)
Francis (Latin)
Franklin (English)
Fraser (English)
Frederick (German)

Thoughts and Feelings...

....
....
....
....
....
....
....
....
....
....
....

tip · tip

THERE ARE
COUNTLESS PLACES TO
LOOK FOR NAME INSPIRATION: TRY
CHECKING OUT THE CREDITS ON TV
SHOWS, PERUSING THE SHELVES OF YOUR
LOCAL BOOKSTORE FOR AUTHOR NAMES,
OR TAKING NOTE OF NAMES OF CHARACTERS IN
YOUR FAVORITE BOOKS.

DIARY DATES: ....

....

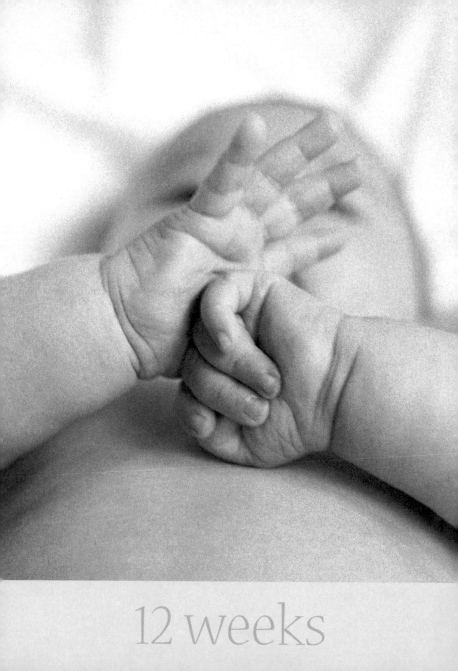

12 weeks

84 days already...

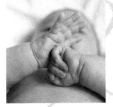

Your Pregnancy

Most pregnant women have their first ultrasound scan at this point. This is an excellent way to determine the progress of the pregnancy, and is your first opportunity to see your growing baby. You will be asked to drink plenty of water before the scan and not to empty your bladder: the extra fluid helps the technician to see the baby. Some hospitals will offer you the option of paying for a photograph of the scanned image.

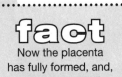

Now the placenta has fully formed, and, around week 12, the risk of miscarriage becomes greatly reduced. Infections also become less of a danger, although rubella is a hazard throughout pregnancy.

Thoughts and Feelings...

....
....
....
....
....
....
....
....
....

DIARY DATES: ....
....

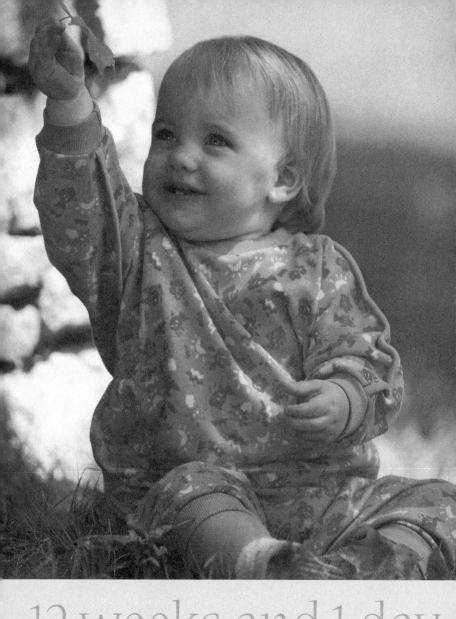

12 weeks and 1 day

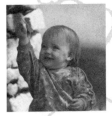

First Scan

At this early stage of the pregnancy the position of the baby is not yet important. Indeed, some babies will be quite active throughout the pregnancy and may be in a different position every time you are checked. Closer to your due date, your care provider will be more concerned if the baby has not turned head down in preparation for the birth. A breech baby is one who is positioned bottom or foot down.

Thoughts and Feelings...

....

....

....

....

....

....

....

....

....

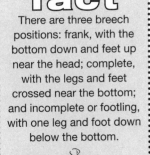

fact

There are three breech positions: frank, with the bottom down and feet up near the head; complete, with the legs and feet crossed near the bottom; and incomplete or footling, with one leg and foot down below the bottom.

DIARY DATES: ....

....

12 weeks and 2 days

day 86

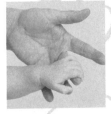

Giving Birth

In the uterus, the membranes form a thin bag that contain the baby and the amniotic fluid. The membranes protect the baby against infections, and the amniotic fluid sees to it that your belly can take a knock without your baby suffering. Your waters break when the membranes of the amniotic sac split and either a gush or a trickle of liquid comes from your vagina.

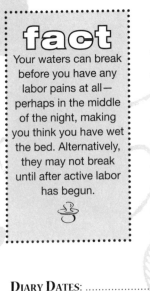

fact

Your waters can break before you have any labor pains at all— perhaps in the middle of the night, making you think you have wet the bed. Alternatively, they may not break until after active labor has begun.

Thoughts and Feelings...

....
....
....
....
....
....
....
....
....

Diary Dates: ....
....

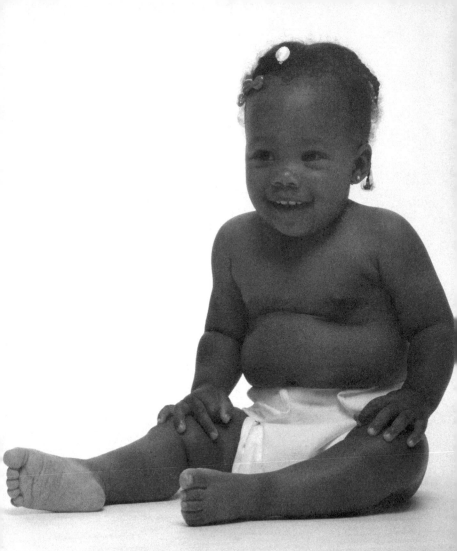

12 weeks and 3 days

day 87

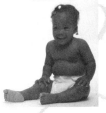

Health and Fitness

Being pregnant changes your metabolism to such an extent that, even when you're resting, you're still using more energy than usual. As a result, pregnant women—from the fourth month on—may feel faint or weak if they don't eat for a while. If you have suffered acute morning sickness, your weight may even have dropped. As you get your appetite back, try to eat regularly and healthily to build up your strength.

Thoughts and Feelings...

....

....

....

....

....

....

....

....

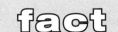

Flatulence, as well as burping, can be an increasing problem during pregnancy. Vegetables that help stop constipation can increase gas. Try eating smaller meals more frequently to reduce the burps.

DIARY DATES: ....

....

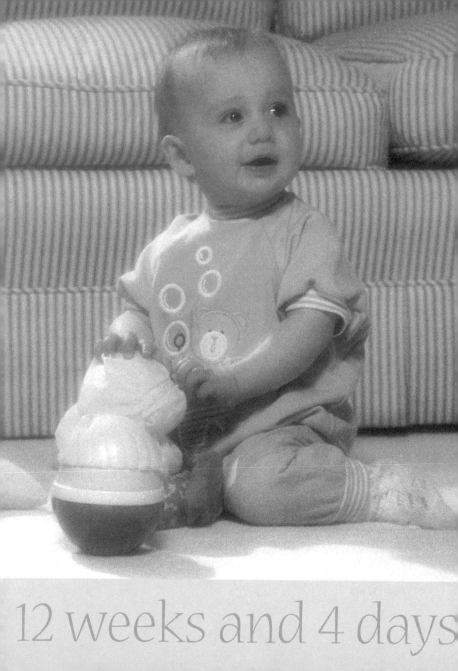

12 weeks and 4 days

day 88

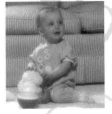

Baby's Development

Basically, the baby is now complete: all the bits and pieces are there. Now the baby just has plenty of growing to do. Her enlarged head accounts for one third of her total length and the tongue, salivary glands and taste buds have formed. The tiny teeth are already present in the gums. Your baby is about 3in (7.5cm) long. The date of delivery can now be adjusted according to these measurements.

fact

You can now hear your baby's heartbeat, and your care provider will check the heartbeat using a fetal stethoscope or a small handheld electrical device. Her heart is beating at between 110 and 160 times per minute.

Thoughts and Feelings...

....
....
....
....
....
....
....
....

DIARY DATES: ....
....

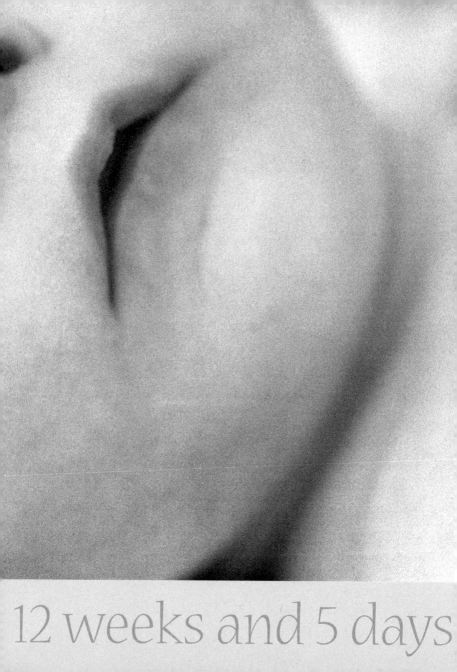

12 weeks and 5 days

day 89

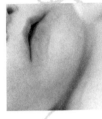

Did You Know?

If you are experiencing pregnancy as a single woman, you may be facing some additional anxieties such as financial, career, and/or custody issues. If at all possible, try to enlist the help and support of a family member or a friend. A birthing partner who will support you right through until the birth of your new baby can give you that much needed sense of support and solidarity.

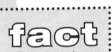

Pregnancy is a joyful time, but it can also bring added pressures to the most solid of relationships. Hormones, fear of the future and financial worries can all add to the mix.

"Stop trying to perfect your child, but keep trying to perfect your relationship with him."

Anonymous

Thoughts and Feelings...

....

....

....

....

....

....

DIARY DATES: ....

....

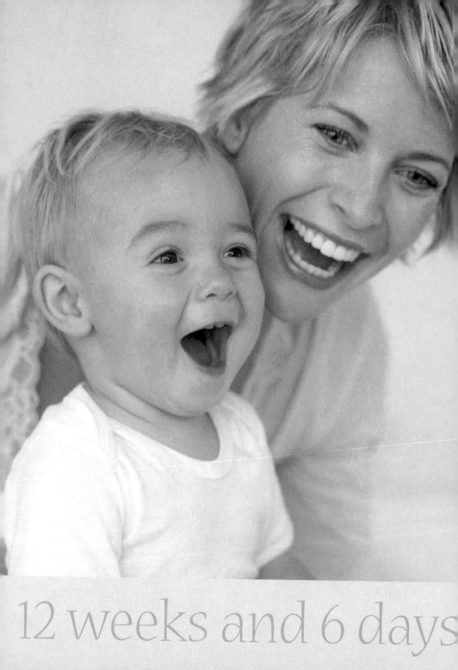

12 weeks and 6 days

day 90

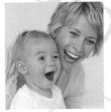

Baby Names for Girls

Gail (Hebrew)
Gay (French)
Gemma (Irish)
Georgia (Latin)
Geraldine (French)
Germaine (French)
Gertrude (German)

Gillian (English)
Gladys (Welsh)
Glenda (Welsh)
Gloria (Latin)
Grace (Latin)
Griselda (German)
Gwyneth (Welsh)

Thoughts and Feelings...

....
....
....
....
....
....
....
....
....
....

tip · tip

THE NATURAL WORLD CAN BE A GREAT SOURCE OF INSPIRATION FOR CHILDREN'S NAMES. FLOWERS, PRECIOUS STONES, RIVERS AND MOUNTAINS CAN ALL BE EXPLORED FOR ORIGINAL NAMES.

DIARY DATES: ....
....

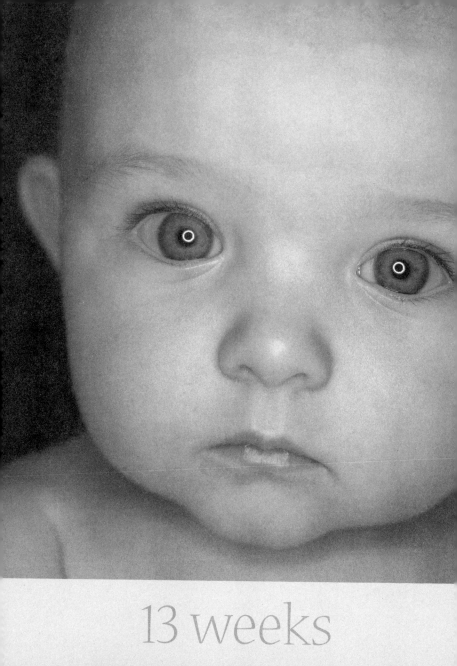

13 weeks

day 91

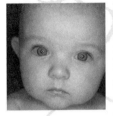

Your Pregnancy

The pregnancy may not yet be visible on the outside although most pregnant women have by now become a bit wider in the waist and around the hips. Pregnancy symptoms that you may now be experiencing could include fatigue, headaches, nasal congestion, increased saliva, tender breasts, nausea, increased urination, and possibly faintness.

Thoughts and Feelings...

....
....
....
....
....
....
....
....
....

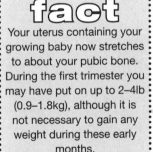

fact
Your uterus containing your growing baby now stretches to about your pubic bone. During the first trimester you may have put on up to 2–4lb (0.9–1.8kg), although it is not necessary to gain any weight during these early months.

DIARY DATES: ....
....

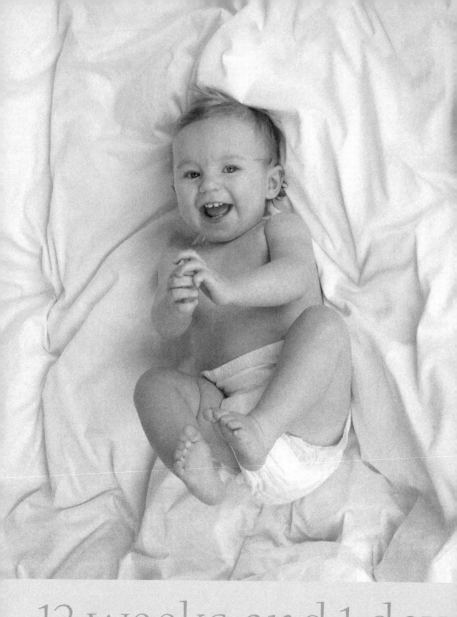

13 weeks and 1 day

day 92

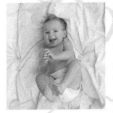

Did You Know?

An amniocentesis test can be taken around week 16. A thin needle is used to take some amniotic fluid via the abdominal wall. The fetal cells from this amniotic fluid are analysed for chromosomal disorders like Down Syndrome or neural tube defects. The physician will use an abdominal ultrasound scan to monitor the exact position of the baby as the needle is inserted. All invasive tests carry a slightly increased risk of miscarriage.

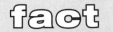

Your care provider may advise you to have an amnio if you are an older woman, your nuchal scan indicated a high risk, family medical history suggests a higher risk, or an ultrasound scan has shown up something that warrants further investigation.

Thoughts and Feelings...

....
....
....
....
....
....
....
....

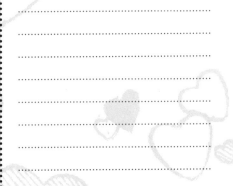

DIARY DATES: ....

....

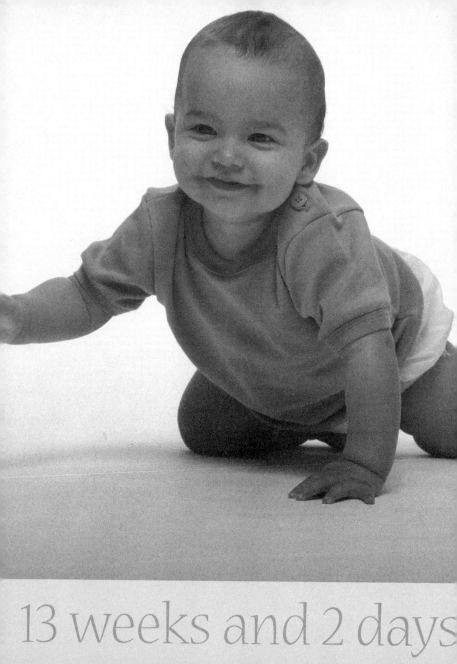

13 weeks and 2 days

day 93

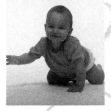

Giving Birth

When your waters break, you need to take note of the color of the liquid. It should be clear, whitish, or pinkish, sometimes there are white flakes floating in it (particles of sebum from the baby) and it smells sweet, as opposed to urine. If it is a bit green or brown, then it contains meconium, the baby's first bowel movement. In this case, alert your care provider immediately.

Thoughts and Feelings...

....

....

....

....

....

....

....

....

....

WARNING

MECONIUM IS A MIXTURE OF AMNIOTIC FLUID, SKIN CELLS AND OTHER FOETAL WASTE THAT MAKES UP THE BABY'S FIRST BOWEL MOVEMENT AND WILL HAVE A DARK, TARRY APPEARANCE. IF THIS HAPPENS IN THE WOMB THE BABY CAN INHALE THE SUBSTANCE AND BECOME DISTRESSED.

DIARY DATES: ....

....

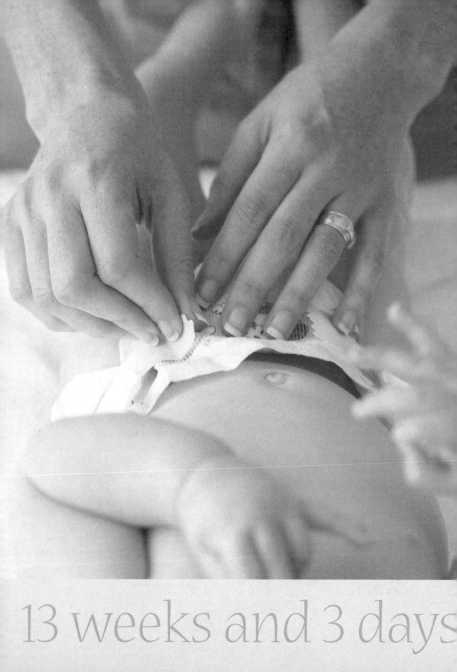

13 weeks and 3 days

day 94

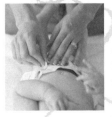

Health and Fitness

Generally speaking, there is no need for special diets during pregnancy: simply eat a varied, balanced diet and ensure a sufficient intake of vitamins and calcium. This is not the time to slim down or embark on a restrictive diet of any kind. To be healthy, you could cut down on sugar—particularly fizzy drinks and snacks—and watch your fat intake from junk food.

WARNING

To avoid health risks, wash vegetables and salads thoroughly. Do not eat raw or undercooked meat or eggs during pregnancy, avoid shellfish, and don't eat food that has gone past its 'sell by' or 'best before' date.

Thoughts and Feelings...

....

....

....

....

....

....

....

....

Diary Dates: ....

....

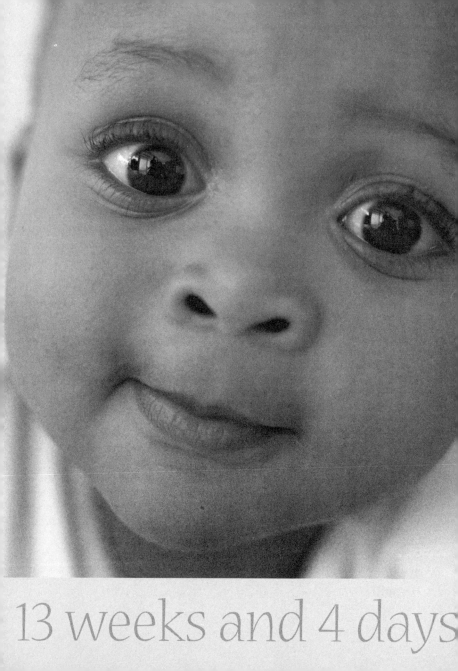

13 weeks and 4 days

day 95

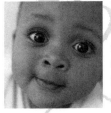

Baby's Development

The baby can now bend his arms at the elbows and the wrist; the fingers can bend and make a fist. The features on the face the nose, chin and forehead, are becoming more defined. Your baby may even be trying out lip movements in preparation for the reflex sucking action that is so crucial to the newborn infant. The fetus is now about 3³/₈in (8.5cm) long.

Thoughts and Feelings...

....
....
....
....
....
....
....
....
....

fact

Blood is pumping around your baby's body then out to the placenta via the umbilical cord, where the waste products (urine and carbon dioxide) are replaced by oxygenated, nutrient-rich blood.

DIARY DATES: ....
....

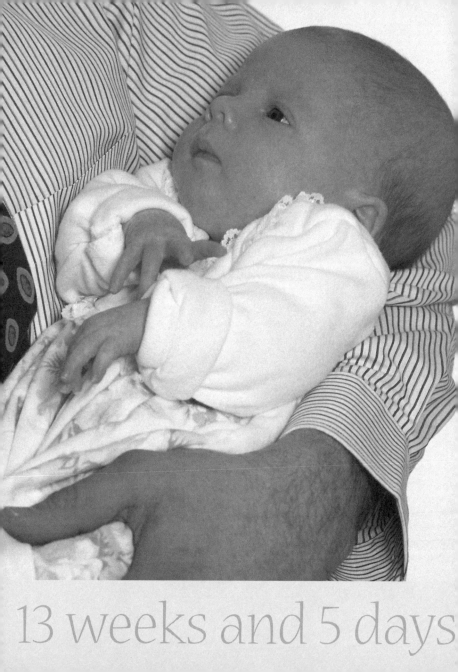

13 weeks and 5 days

day 96

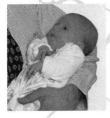

Did You Know?

"I've done it once by sticking to the rules; the sleepless nights, vomit and endless amounts of dirty diapers. I just wanted to enjoy my second child so that's what I did. I gave myself a nanny as a present to do all the dirty work so I could get some joy and relaxation out of it. I don't want the strain and stress of calming a crying baby anymore. I think everybody feels the same about this. It's just that those who can't afford a nanny are quicker to judge you."

Priscilla Presley, actress (taken from *Beau Monde*)

Thoughts and Feelings...

....
....
....
....
....
....

DIARY DATES: ....

....

tip · tip · tip · tip · tip · tip · tip · tip · tip · tip · tip · tip · tip · tip · tip · tip

CAN'T AFFORD HELP? NOW IS THE TIME TO TAKE UP OFFERS OF HELP FROM FRIENDS, FAMILY AND NEIGHBOURS. DRAW UP A LIST OF WHAT YOU NEED—INCLUDING MEALS—THEN PUT IN YOUR REQUESTS. IF YOU AND YOUR PARTNER AGREE, ASKING SOMEONE YOU TRUST TO COME AND STAY FOR THE FIRST COUPLE OF WEEKS CAN BE REWARDING.

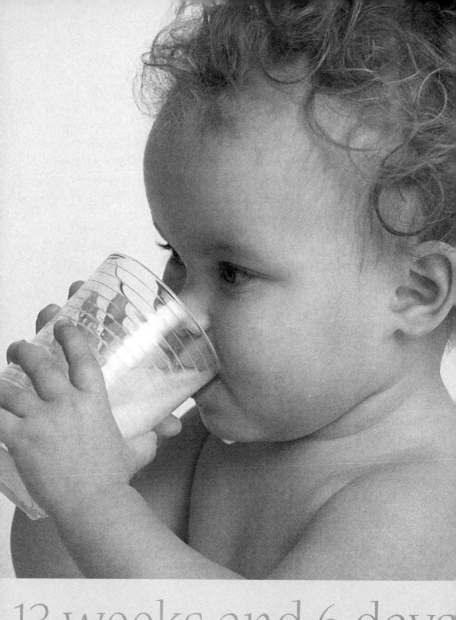

13 weeks and 6 days

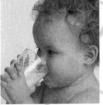

Baby Names for Boys

Gabriel (Hebrew)
Galbraith (Irish)
Garfield (English)
Garrett (Irish)
Garth (English)
Gary (English)
Gavin (Welsh)
Gene (English)
Geoffrey (German)
George (Greek)

Gerald (German)
Gilbert (German)
Glen (Irish)
Godfrey (German)
Godwin (English)
Gordon (English)
Graham (English)
Gregory (Greek)
Guy (French)

Thoughts and Feelings...

....
....
....
....
....
....
....
....
....

WARNING

THE NAME OF YOUR FAVORITE CELEBRITY OR SPORTING HERO IS OFTEN TEMPTING AS A CHOICE FOR YOUR NEW BABY; BE WARNED, HOWEVER, THAT CELEBRITIES CAN GO OUT OF FASHION AND THEIR NAMES GO ALONG WITH THEM.

DIARY DATES: ....

....

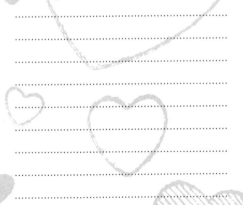

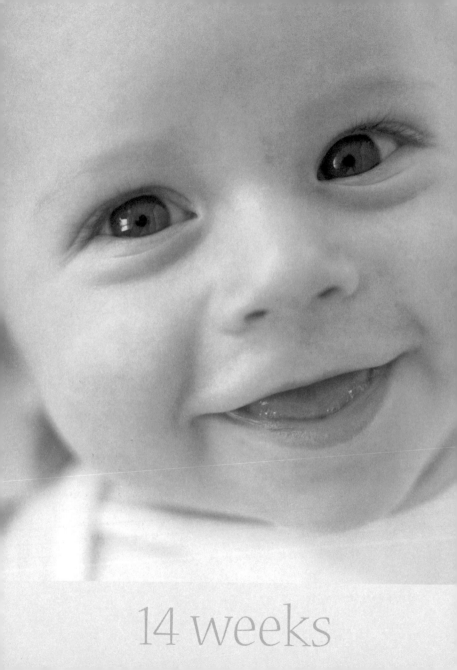

14 weeks

14 weeks

day 98

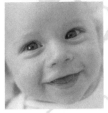

Your Pregnancy

The ultrasound scan picture is obtained by passing a hand-held wand called a transducer over your abdomen. The wand emits high-frequency sound waves that bounce off the solid form of your baby and send back an image to a computer screen. Before the technician begins, they will apply a thick layer of jelly on your abdomen to enable the wand to run smoothly.

Thoughts and Feelings...

WARNING

DEPENDING ON THE COOPERATION OF THE BABY—IN OTHER WORDS HOW HE IS LYING—THE TECHNICIAN MAY BE ABLE TO IDENTIFY THE SEX OF YOUR BABY. ASK ABOUT THIS IF YOU WOULD LIKE TO KNOW, AND BE SURE TO LET THEM KNOW YOU'RE NOT INTERESTED IF YOU PREFER THIS TO BE A SURPRISE AT THE BIRTH.

....
....
....
....
....
....
....
....
....
....

DIARY DATES: Routine prenatal blood test and discussion on optional tests

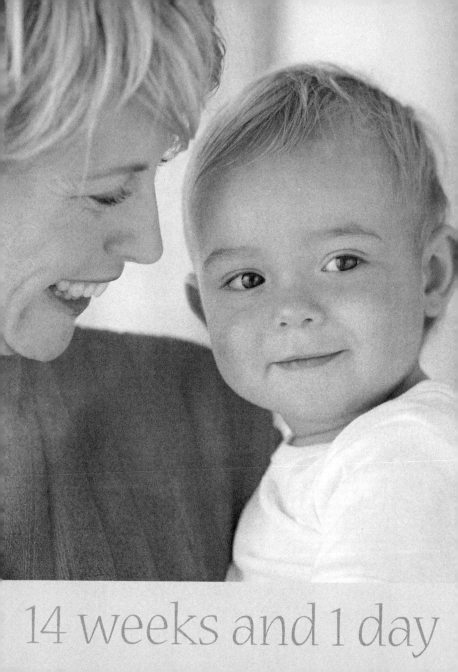

14 weeks and 1 day

day 99

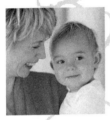

Did You Know?

Ultrasound scans can be used to check on any abnormal developments in your growing baby. A series of measurements will be taken each time you have a scan and they can be used to calculate the growth and organ development of the fetus. If you have a higher risk pregnancy, such as a multiple birth, it is likely you will be scanned more frequently throughout your pregnancy.

Thoughts and Feelings...

....
....
....
....
....
....
....
....
....

tip · tip

SOME CARE PROVIDERS WILL SCAN AT AN EARLY APPOINTMENT AND AGAIN AT 20 WEEKS. SOME WILL ONLY SCAN ONCE. IF YOU ARE PARTICULARLY CONCERNED FOR THE WELL-BEING OF YOUR BABY, YOU CAN REQUEST A SCAN, AND, YOUR CARE PROVIDER MAY AGREE.

DIARY DATES: ....
....

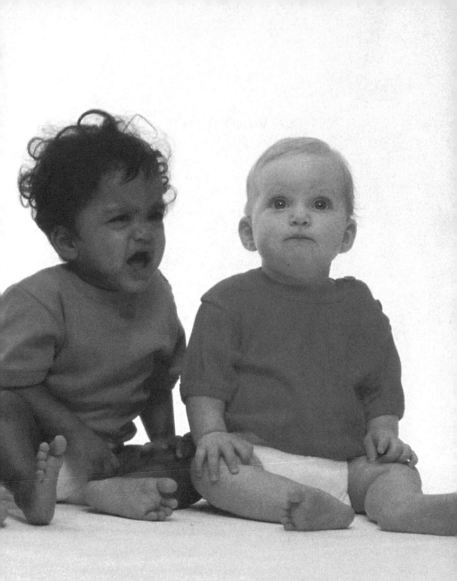

14 weeks and 2 days

day 100

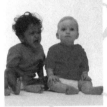

Giving Birth

It is difficult to imagine exactly what a contraction (labor pain) feels like if you've never had one. It is comparable with menstrual cramps, because the womb also contracts during the menstrual period. Menstrual cramps, however, are often lengthy and nagging whereas contractions have a clear beginning and end. They come and go like waves.

Thoughts and Feelings...

....

....

....

....

....

....

....

....

tip · tip

BREAST AND NIPPLE STIMULATION IN LATE PREGNANCY CAN PRODUCE QUITE STRONG CONTRACTIONS. IT IS EVEN POSSIBLE TO RESTART A STALLED LABOR BY THIS METHOD—SOMETHING YOU AND OUR PARTNER MAY WANT TO CONSIDER.

DIARY DATES: ....

....

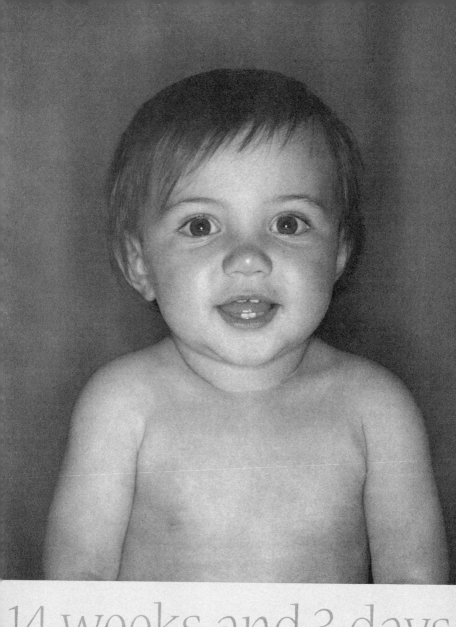

14 weeks and 3 days

day 101

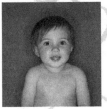

Health and Fitness

While you are pregnant you should avoid certain foods that carry an increased risk of Listeria infections (also known as listeriosis). This extremely violent infection produces symptoms similar to influenza or meningitis and can cause miscarriage. Avoid unpasteurized milk and products made from unpasteurized milk—such as soft cheeses, blue-vein cheeses, and cheese made from goat or sheep milk. Also avoid pâtés, soft ice cream, and prepared, bagged salads.

Thoughts and Feelings...

....
....
....
....
....
....
....
....

WARNING

LISTERIOSIS CAN ALSO BE CONTRACTED BY DIRECT CONTACT WITH INFECTED ANIMALS. YOU SHOULD HAVE AN INCREASED AWARENESS OF PERSONAL AND KITCHEN HYGIENE DURING PREGNANCY TO MINIMIZE THE RISKS OF FOOD POISONING IN GENERAL.

DIARY DATES: ....
....

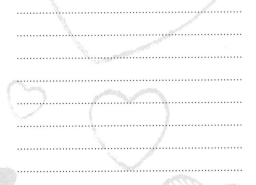

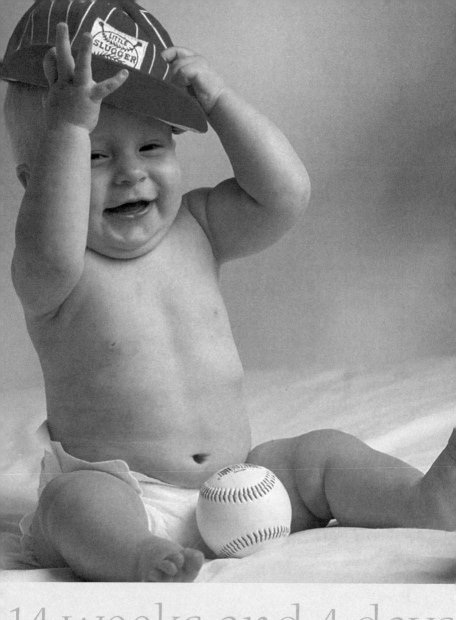
14 weeks and 4 days

day 102

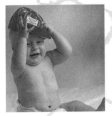

Baby's Development

The taste organs are now developing: the fetus recognizes the taste of the amniotic fluid it is in and takes it in through the skin and by swallowing it. Hair is growing not only on the baby's head, but also as eyebrows and even eyelashes. The baby starts to lose her top-heavy look as her overall height increases: the legs are now longer than the arms. Baby is 4³⁄₈in (11cm) in length.

Thoughts and Feelings...

....

....

....

....

....

....

....

....

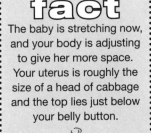

fact

The baby is stretching now, and your body is adjusting to give her more space. Your uterus is roughly the size of a head of cabbage and the top lies just below your belly button.

DIARY DATES: ....

....

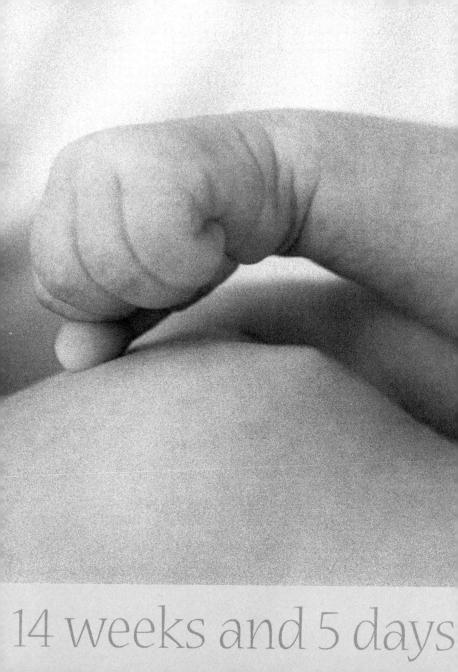

14 weeks and 5 days

day 103

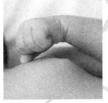

Did You Know?

It is possible to settle your newborn baby straight into his crib, but a small, cozy bassinet or "Moses basket" may help to make him feel secure—having just left the confined comfort of your womb. It also makes moving the new baby from room to room without disturbing him very easy, plus if you feel the need to have this delicate new arrival close by, you can place the basket close to your bed at night.

"To understand your parents' love you must raise children yourself."

Chinese proverb

Thoughts and Feelings...

....

....

....

....

....

....

....

WARNING

IF YOU ARE A LIGHT SLEEPER, YOU MIGHT FIND THE SNUFFLING, HICCOUGHING AND SNORING OF YOUR NEW ARRIVAL IS KEEPING YOU FROM YOUR PRECIOUS SLEEP. INVEST IN A BABY MONITOR AND MOVE BABY INTO ANOTHER ROOM.

DIARY DATES: ....

....

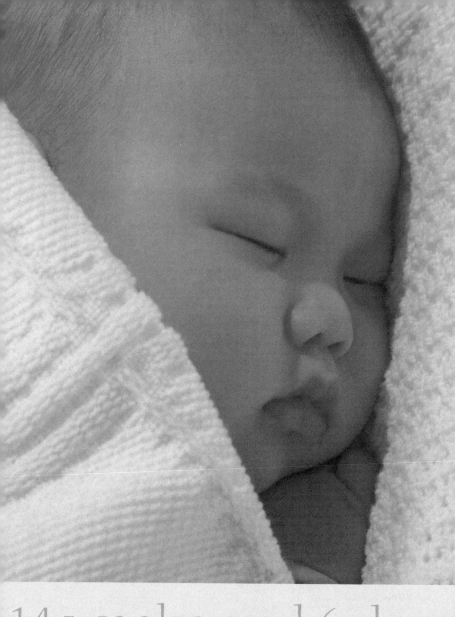

14 weeks and 6 days

day 104

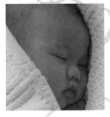

Baby Names for Girls

Hannah (Hebrew)	Hermia (Greek)
Harriet (German)	Hester (Greek)
Hazel (English)	Hilary (Greek)
Heather (English)	Holly (English)
Helen (Greek)	Hortense (Latin)
Henrietta (German)	Hyacinth (Greek)

Thoughts and Feelings…

....

....

....

....

....

....

....

....

....

....

....

fact

Most likely the longest name for a person is Rhoshandiatellyneshiaunn-eveshenk Koyaanfsquatsiuty Williams, daughter of Mr. and Mrs. James L. Williams from Beaumont, Texas born on September 12, 1984. In October 1984, her father submitted a proposal, in which his daughter's first name was extended to 1019 letters and her second name to 36 letters. (*Guinness Book of Records*)

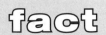

DIARY DATES: ....

....

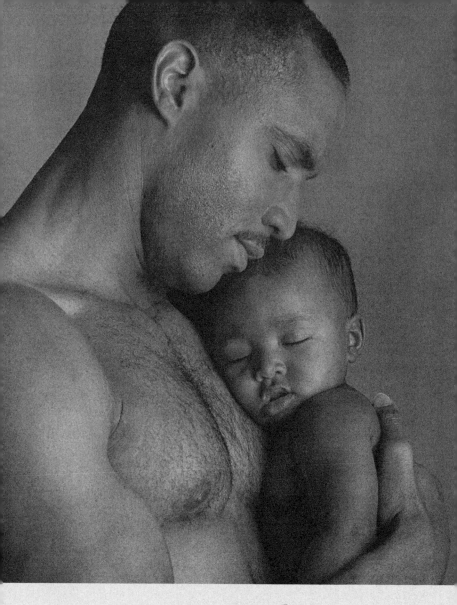

15 weeks

15 weeks

day 105

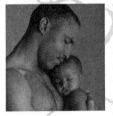

Your Pregnancy

Whether or not to have invasive tests such as amniocentesis or chorionic villus sampling (CVS) is a decision only you and the father of your baby can take. There is a slightly increased risk of miscarriage with both procedures. CVS happens at 11 weeks but is less accurate than an amnio. The results from an amnio will usually not be available until your 20th week of pregnancy.

Thoughts and Feelings...

....
....
....
....
....
....
....
....
....

reminder

Only you can decide what steps to take if your baby is found to have a problem. You may wish to terminate, the pregnancy or you may want to prepare ahead for the birth of a child with special needs.

DIARY DATES: ....
....

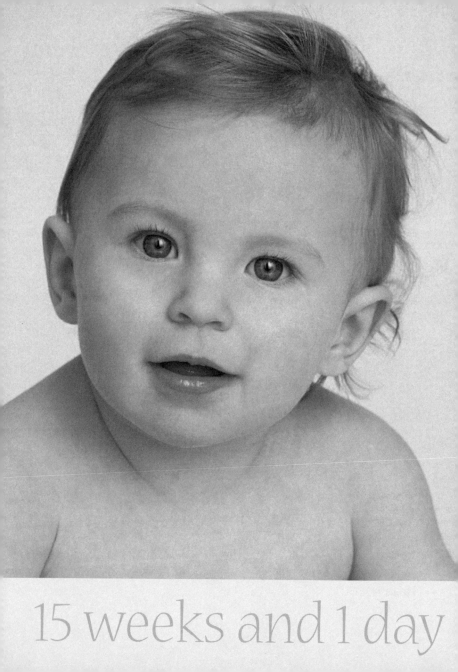

15 weeks and 1 day

day 106

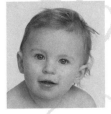

Did You Know?

At birth your baby's eyesight may be a little blurred, but he can focus on objects held about 8in (20cm) away from his face. He will be particularly fascinated by objects that move, and there is a good chance that he can make out colours. Babies are also born with several reflex actions, but blinking is the only one that they will keep for life.

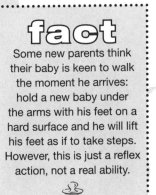

fact

Some new parents think their baby is keen to walk the moment he arrives: hold a new baby under the arms with his feet on a hard surface and he will lift his feet as if to take steps. However, this is just a reflex action, not a real ability.

Thoughts and Feelings...

....
....
....
....
....
....
....
....
....
....

DIARY DATES: ....
....

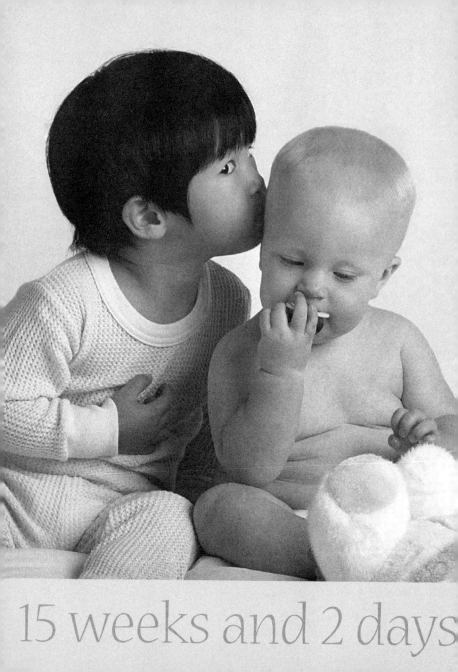

15 weeks and 2 days

day 107

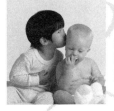

Giving Birth

No matter how enthusiastically you may start giving birth, there will undoubtedly be moments when you think you can no longer cope, times when you'll be tired and extremely irritable. You may have moments of fear, doubt, frustration, and uncertainty. It's all part of giving birth and although it is hugely challenging, this is the most rewarding work you will ever do.

Thoughts and Feelings...

....

....

....

....

....

....

....

....

....

tip · tip

HOWEVER MUCH RESEARCH YOU DO, HOWEVER MANY PEOPLE YOU TALK TO, IT IS HARD TO PREPARE FOR CHILDBIRTH. ULTIMATELY YOUR EXPERIENCE WILL BE UNIQUE; BE OPEN MINDED AND ABOVE ALL FOLLOW YOUR OWN PATH.

DIARY DATES: ....

....

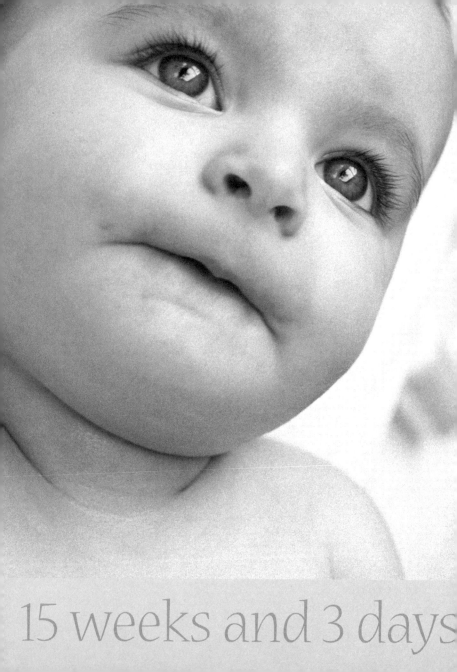

15 weeks and 3 days

day 108

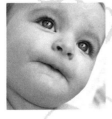

Health and Fitness

Physical exercise during pregnancy is mainly a question of common sense and listening to your body if it tells you it is straining. You know your own body best, both during the pregnancy and after it. Only you can judge what you find pleasant and what is a burden. Always avoid contact sports or one where you or the baby could be hit, and always check with your doctor before taking up a new exercise.

Thoughts and Feelings...

....
....
....
....
....
....
....
....
....

WARNING

STOP ANY EXERCISE IMMEDIATELY IF YOU EXPERIENCE DIZZINESS, SEVERE HEADACHES, VAGINAL BLEEDING, ABDOMINAL OR CHEST PAINS, OR EXTREME SHORTNESS OF BREATH. SEEK MEDICAL ADVICE IF YOU ARE AT ALL WORRIED.

DIARY DATES: ....
....

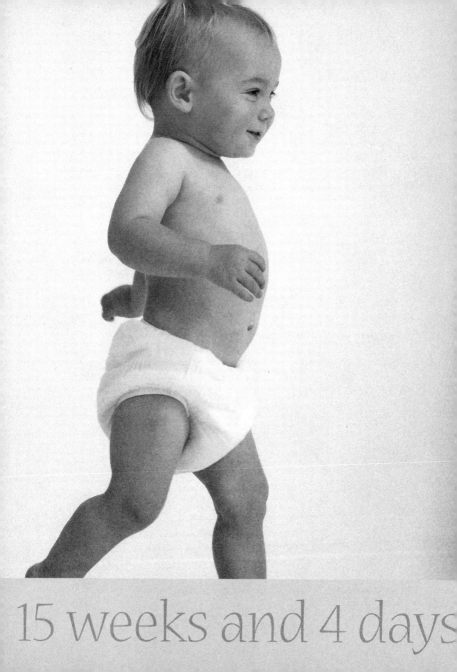

15 weeks and 4 days

day 109

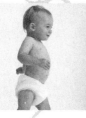

Baby's Development

The movements of the fetus are becoming more acrobatic but you probably still won't be able to feel them. A growth of hair (also known as first hair, down, or lanugo) covers the whole body; this is thought to maintain the right body temperature. The skeleton is developing as cartilage is replaced with a soft spongy, woven bone. The baby is now about 6in (15cm) long.

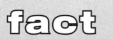

fact

The placenta is about 3in (7.5cm) in diameter and the umbilical cord attaching it to the fetus is about as long as the baby. The cord will continue to grow as the baby grows, and it is crucial for delivering nutrients from the placenta.

Thoughts and Feelings...

....

....

....

....

....

....

....

....

....

DIARY DATES: ....

....

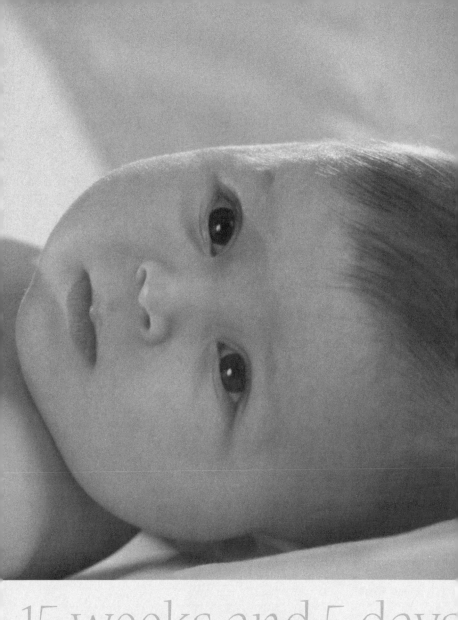

15 weeks and 5 days

day 110

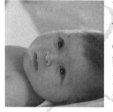

Did You Know?

You may find that everyone has an opinion on whether you are having a boy or a girl based on how you are carrying your baby. However, where your baby lies in your belly is entirely based on your build, your posture, and your pregnancy history. If you have had previous pregnancies then your abdominal muscles will be more relaxed and it is likely you will be carrying your baby lower.

"Every child is an artist. The problem is to remain an artist once they grow up."

Pablo Picasso, artist (1881–1973)

Thoughts and Feelings...

....
....
....
....
....
....

tip · tip

START FINDING OUT ABOUT BABY AND TODDLER GROUPS IN YOUR NEIGHBORHOOD. TALK TO OTHER MOTHERS; CHECK OUT NOTICEBOARDS AT YOUR CARE PROVIDER'S OFFICE OR LIBRARY. YOUR BABY WILL ENJOY THE COMPANY OF HIS OR HER PEERS FROM A SURPRISINGLY YOUNG AGE, AND YOU WILL MEET OTHER MOMS.

DIARY DATES: ....
....

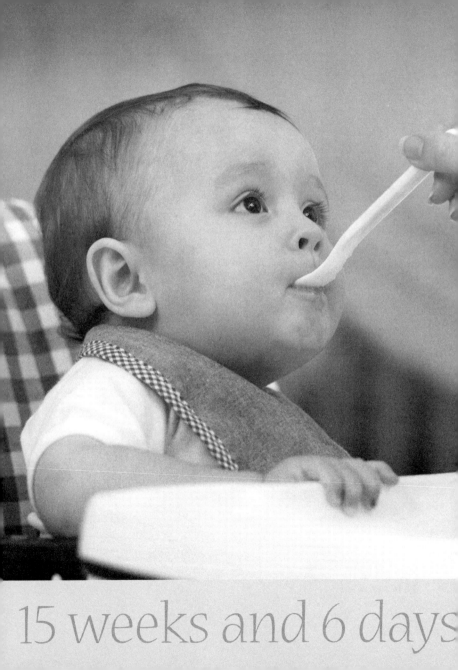

15 weeks and 6 days

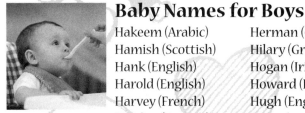

Baby Names for Boys

Hakeem (Arabic)
Hamish (Scottish)
Hank (English)
Harold (English)
Harvey (French)
Hayden (English)
Henry (German)

Herman (German)
Hilary (Greek)
Hogan (Irish)
Howard (English)
Hugh (English)
Humphrey (English)

WARNING

WHEN CHOOSING YOUR BABY'S NAME, REMEMBER TO SOUND IT OUT WITH YOUR LAST NAME AS WELL. YOU MAY BE DISMAYED TO DISCOVER AN ODD RHYME, ALLITERATION OR ONOMATOPOEIA WHEN YOU SAY THE NAMES TOGETHER OUT LOUD.

Thoughts and Feelings...

....
....
....
....
....
....
....
....

DIARY DATES: ....

....

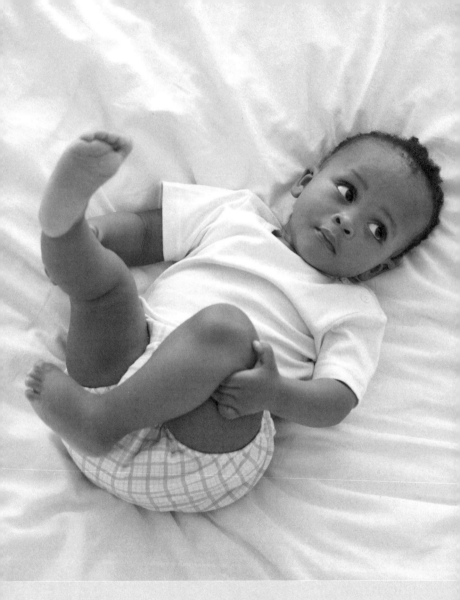
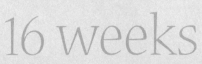
16 weeks

day 112

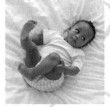

Your Pregnancy

If you suffered a lot from nausea and other pregnancy conditions in the early months you have probably entered a better period by now. Your body has gradually adjusted to the pregnancy and most mothers-to-be feel very well between the fourth and seventh month. This is the time for you and your partner to plan a final peaceful holiday – or even to go with your first child, as life will be more hectic after the new arrival.

Thoughts and Feelings...

....
....
....
....
....
....
....
....

tip · tip

CRAMPS ARE ANOTHER SYMPTOM OF PREGNANCY—ESPECIALLY IN THE CALF MUSCLES AND FEET. THEY CAN COME ON VERY SUDDENLY, PARTICULARLY AT NIGHT IN BED. TRY PULLING YOUR TOES UP TOWARDS YOUR ANKLES AND MASSAGING THE AFFECTED MUSCLES.

DIARY DATES: Routine check-up
....

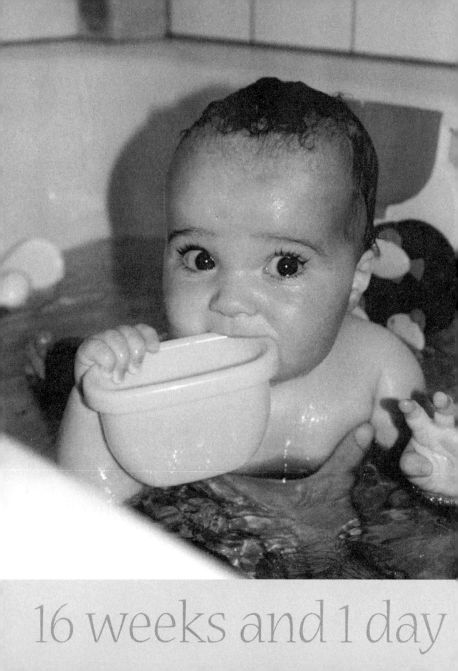

16 weeks and 1 day

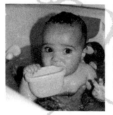

Did You Know?

A midwife is an expert in dealing with pregnancy and childbirth but he or she is restricted in the medical procedures they may carry out and the prescription of medicine. you may choose to have a midwife assist you with your birth, but if your pregnancy has complications (such as a multiple birth, a difficult pregnancy in the past, or you are an older mom-to-be, then you may may also require the care of an obstetrician or other medical doctor

Thoughts and Feelings...

....
....
....
....
....
....
....
....

reminder

If you are expecting twins (or more), the best people to talk to about the experience is other moms of multiples. Look for a club or support group for parents of multiples on the Web or in your local newspaper.

DIARY DATES: ....

....

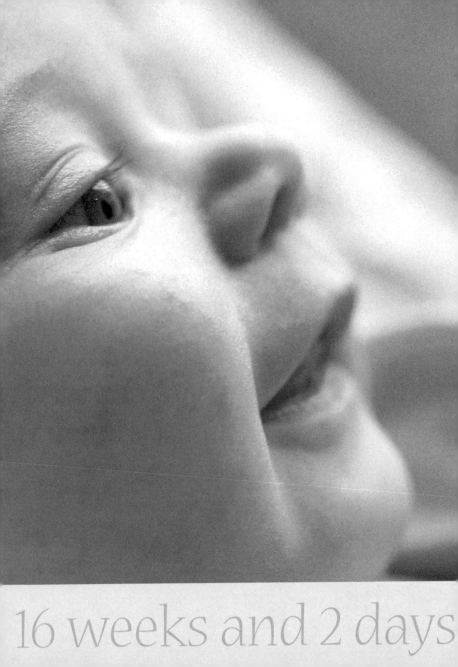

16 weeks and 2 days

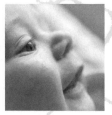

Giving Birth

Back pains during childbirth can be associated with contractions or they may also be a completely separate issue. Ideally the baby will position itself with its back against your abdomen for delivery, but if it lies with its back towards your back in an 'occipito posterior' position it will cause you extreme backache during labour, and may delay delivery. You can still have a natural birth, but the baby will arrive face up.

Thoughts and Feelings...

....
....
....
....
....
....
....
....
....
....

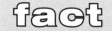

fact

Contractions may start at 20–45 minutes apart. Closer to delivery they will be just minutes apart and be much more intense. Walking or moving around may increase the intensity of your contractions.

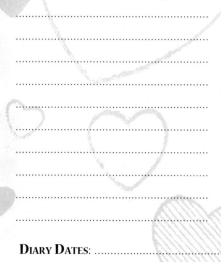

DIARY DATES: ....
....

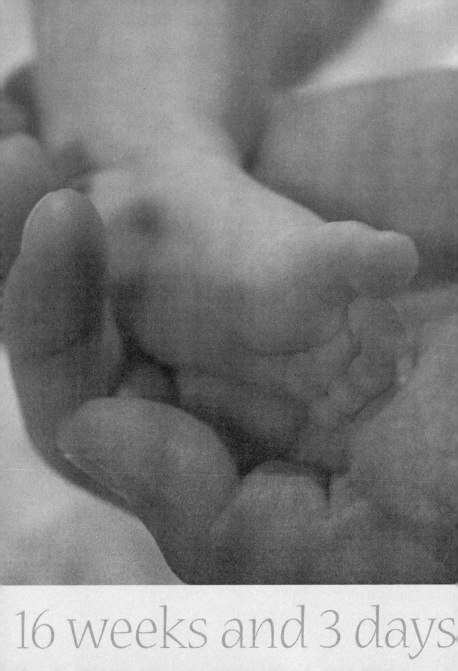

16 weeks and 3 days

day 115

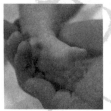

Health and Fitness

You can use physical exercise to strengthen the muscles that carry the extra weight of the enlarged womb and the baby, especially the legs, lower back, stomach muscles and feet. Some movements, however—such as lying on the ground and raising your legs while keeping them stretched or sit-ups— place an unnecessarily heavy burden on the muscles, which have a lot to deal with as it is.

Thoughts and Feelings...

....

....

....

....

....

....

....

....

....

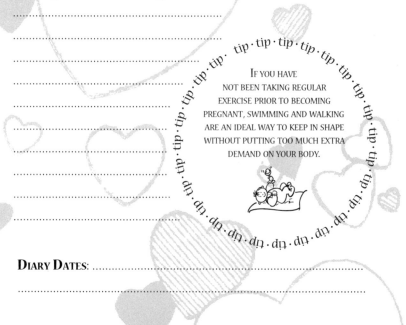

tip · tip

IF YOU HAVE NOT BEEN TAKING REGULAR EXERCISE PRIOR TO BECOMING PREGNANT, SWIMMING AND WALKING ARE AN IDEAL WAY TO KEEP IN SHAPE WITHOUT PUTTING TOO MUCH EXTRA DEMAND ON YOUR BODY.

DIARY DATES: ....

....

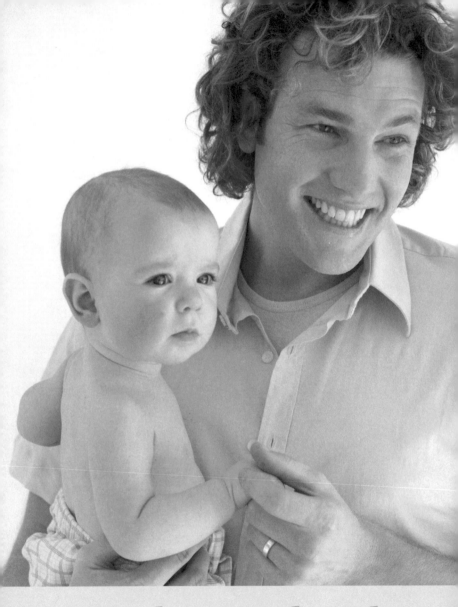

16 weeks and 4 days

day 116

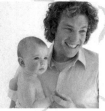

Baby's Development

Your baby's skin is becoming thicker but remains transparent; as a result, the blood vessels are clearly visible. The hair on her head is growing. The muscles are becoming stronger and her movements more powerful. She is moving her limbs and can easily clench and unclench her fists. She is about 7$\frac{1}{8}$ in (18cm) in length.

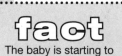

The baby is starting to add weight now as she deposits pockets of brown fat just under the skin. The fat is crucial for the newborn baby to be able to control its body temperature in the outside world.

Thoughts and Feelings...

....
....
....
....
....
....
....
....
....
....

DIARY DATES: ....

....

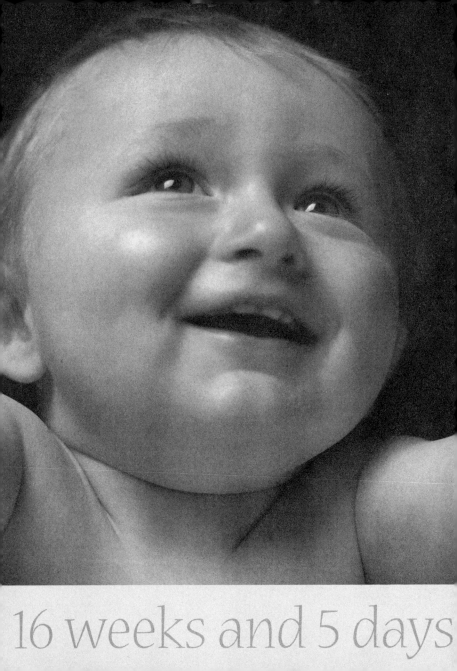

16 weeks and 5 days

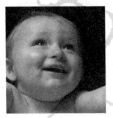

Did You Know?

The average baby can get through up to 50 to 80 diapers a week. Over a year, the cost of diapers is certainly going to mount up. It is still early to be buying baby equipment, but you may want to take a trip to the baby department of a local store. You will be amazed at the equipment you may find yourself purchasing for just the first three to four months of your baby's life!

"Live so that when your children think of fairness and integrity, they think of you."

H. Jackson Brown Jr., American author of the *Life's Little Instruction Book* series

Thoughts and Feelings…

....

....

....

....

....

remember

Planning to give up work when your baby arrives? Now is the time to work out your budget. Note down your expenses now and then consider how things will be if you lose a salary, or if you decide to pay for childcare.

DIARY DATES: ....

....

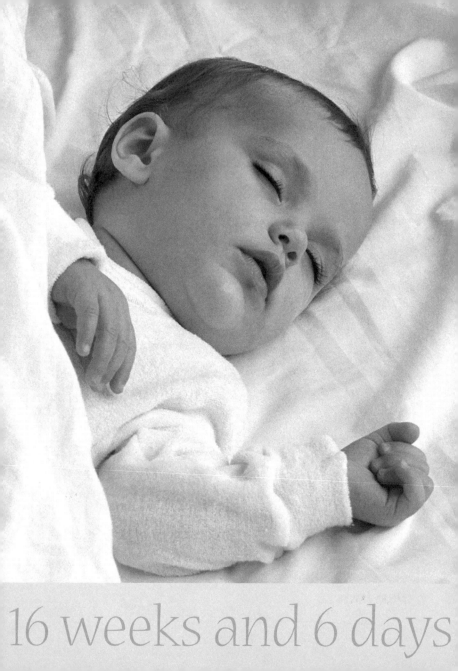

16 weeks and 6 days

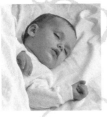

Baby Names for Girls

Ida (English)
Ilana (Hebrew)
Ilse (German)
Imelda (Italian)
Imogen (Latin)
Ingrid (Scandinavian)

Iola (Welsh)
Iona (Greek)
Irene (Greek)
Iris (Greek)
Isabel (Spanish)
Isadora (Latin)
Ivy (English)

Thoughts and Feelings...

....
....
....
....
....
....
....
....
....
....

tip · tip · tip · tip · tip · tip · tip · tip · tip · tip · tip · tip · tip · tip · tip · tip · tip · tip · tip · tip

FOR MANY PEOPLE RELIGION CAN PLAY A LARGE PART IN CHOOSING A NAME. SAINTS' NAMES ARE ALWAYS POPULAR. YOUR TOWN OR REGION MAY HAVE A PATRON SAINT OR YOU MAY CHOOSE THE SAINT OF YOUR PROFESSION— OR SIMPLY A SAINT WHOSE NAME YOU LIKE!

DIARY DATES: ....
....

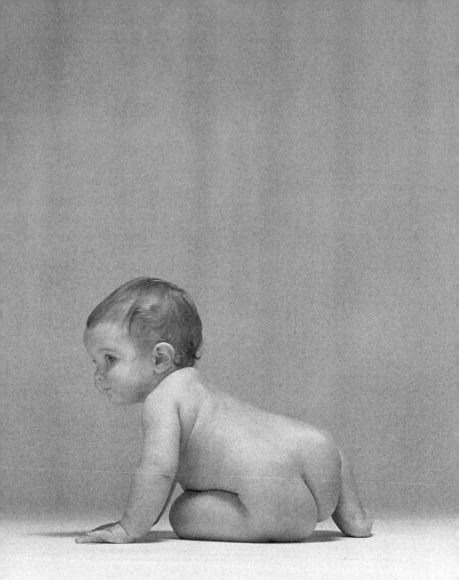

17 weeks

17 weeks

day 119

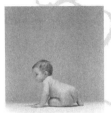

Your Pregnancy

Many women who are experiencing their first pregnancy regularly have short periods of being terror stricken. If you and your partner have only had yourselves to worry about up to this point, it is probably hard to imagine the total change that is about to take over your lives. Luckily, it will be an immensely rewarding transition as well, and one that you will all grow into together once your baby has arrived.

Thoughts and Feelings...

....
....
....
....
....
....
....
....
....

remember

If the arrival of a new baby seems overwhelming, remember that this total dependence on you is only temporary. You will get your life back, and you won't have to wait until your children reach adolescence to regain some freedom.

DIARY DATES: ....
....

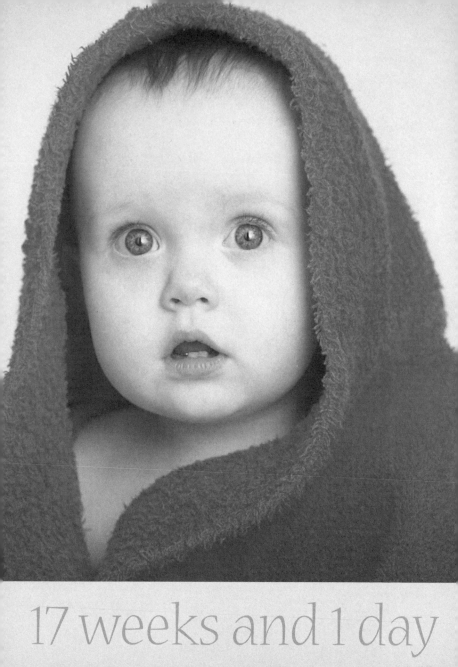

17 weeks and 1 day

day 120

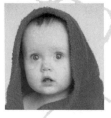

Did You Know?

At around 20 weeks you may go for a screening ultrasound scan. This is an extensive scan that examines the fetal anatomy carefully. The baby's organs are checked one by one and measurements taken. If anything problematic is noted you may still be referred to take an amniocentesis test, even though it is now quite late in your pregnancy.

Thoughts and Feelings...

....

....

....

....

....

....

....

....

....

remember

It is important to choose the right bra during your pregnancy; it is possible your breasts will increase by two sizes during this period, and support is vital to stop breasts sagging. Avoid underwired bras during pregnancy.

DIARY DATES: ....

....

17 weeks and 2 days

day 121

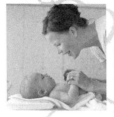

Giving Birth

Try to remember at the start of a contraction that this one, too, will end—and that each contraction takes you a little bit closer to the arrival of your baby. You'll notice that this way the pain becomes more bearable and that you have better control over your body. Once contractions have started there is no need to rush to hospital, but do try to have someone with you.

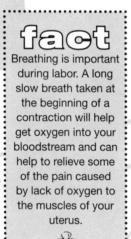

fact

Breathing is important during labor. A long slow breath taken at the beginning of a contraction will help get oxygen into your bloodstream and can help to relieve some of the pain caused by lack of oxygen to the muscles of your uterus.

Thoughts and Feelings...

....

....

....

....

....

....

....

....

DIARY DATES: ....

....

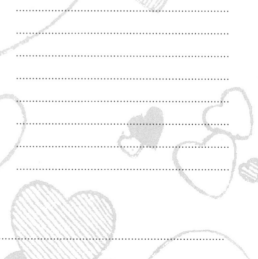

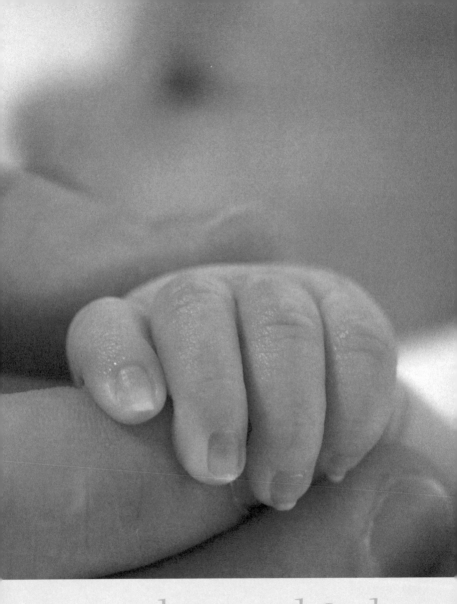

17 weeks and 3 days

day 122

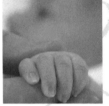

Health and Fitness

The skin, especially on your face, requires special care during pregnancy. Be alert because your skin type may change—from greasy skin to normal or from normal to dry. After a shower or bath, moisturize your skin well. Your body may develop stretch marks as you put on weight; there is nothing you can do to avoid this but moisturizing your stomach with oil or cream will avoid your skin drying out.

Thoughts and Feelings...

....

....

....

....

....

....

....

....

....

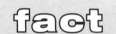

Fluid retention can be a problem during pregnancy, and this can lead to puffiness around the eyes. There is no cure except to rest as much as possible, and if you keep your legs up you will minimize puffy legs and ankles.

DIARY DATES: ....

....

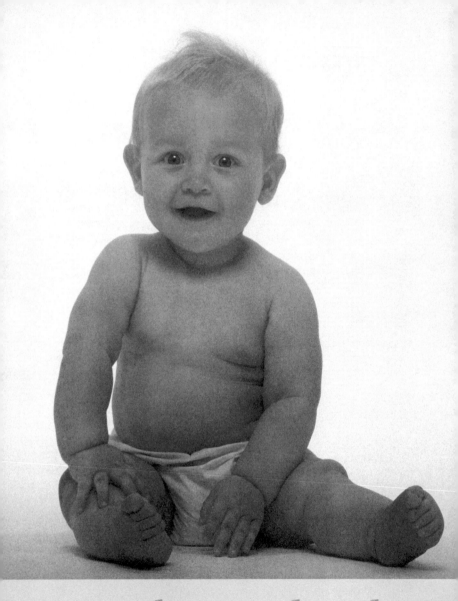

17 weeks and 4 days

day 123

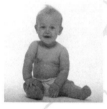

Baby's Development

The baby has just started to be able to distinguish between light and dark through his eyelids; the environment he sees is the amniotic fluid, the womb, and the abdominal wall. The skin is still very wrinkled and will remain so until your baby starts to store up body fat. The baby is about 8in (20cm) long and weighs about 8oz (235g).

Thoughts and Feelings...

....
....
....
....
....
....
....
....
....
....

fact

As the baby becomes bigger and more active, it is likely that you will start to feel your baby moving now. If this is a second pregnancy, and the sensation was familiar, you may have been alert to these movements earlier.

DIARY DATES: ....

....

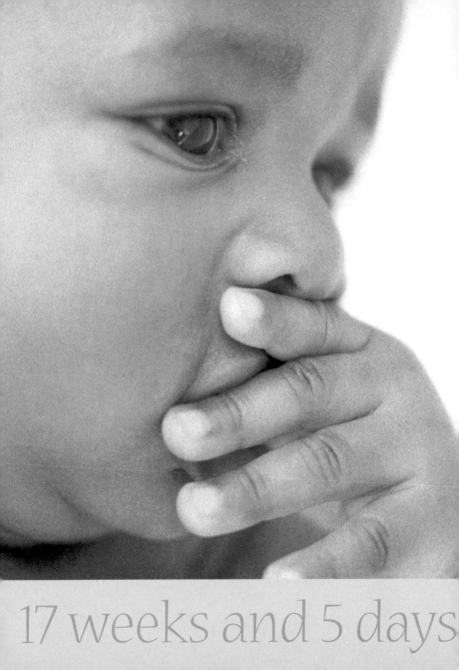

17 weeks and 5 days

day 124

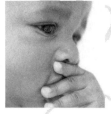

Did You Know?

It is important to learn how to relax deeply during your pregnancy. It will help you to rest and be good for your baby as well. Practise meditative techniques at home or listen to relaxation tapes, or treat yourself to a massage. Be aware, however, that some aromatherapy oils are dangerous during pregnancy, so always consult a trained aromatherapy masseuse.

Thoughts and Feelings...

....

....

....

....

....

....

....

....

....

....

"I'm already looking forward to playing with the children and getting completely filthy with them. I don't trust mothers of young children who always look perfectly groomed. They haven't been with their children; they've been to the beauty salon and the hairdressers instead."

Catherine Zeta-Jones, actress

DIARY DATES: ....

....

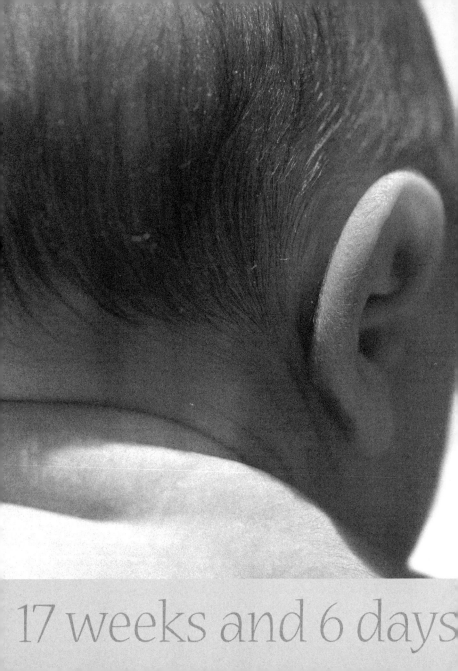

17 weeks and 6 days

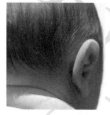

Baby Names for Boys

Ian (Scottish)
Ignatius (English)
Ike (English)
Ilya (Russian)
Imran (Arabic)
Innes (Scottish)

Ira (Hebrew)
Irvin (Scottish)
Irving (English)
Isaac (Hebrew)
Ivan (Czech)

Thoughts and Feelings...

....

....

....

....

....

....

....

....

....

....

....

reminder

Tiny babies grow up to big boys and then full-grown men. If you start off using a cute shortened version of their name or some totally unrelated nickname, you may, horrifyingly, find yourself still using this name when your child is an adult. They won't thank you for it!

DIARY DATES: ....

....

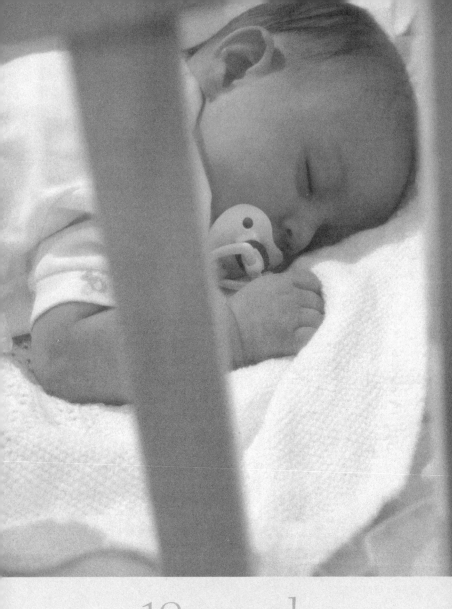

18 weeks

18 weeks

day 126

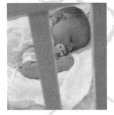

Your Pregnancy

Between the 16th and the 20th week the midwife can feel whether you are expecting twins, or it will show up on your scan. Full term for a twin pregnancy is 38 weeks—not 40 as for a single baby. If you are expecting triplets the date will be brought forward again to 35 weeks and quads are expected by 34 weeks. Premature birth is by far the greatest risk in a multiple pregnancy.

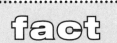

Another risk in multiple births where the babies share the same amniotic sac is twisting or knotting of the umbilical cord. Frequent ultrasound scanning will likely be used to monitor your progress.

Thoughts and Feelings...

....

....

....

....

....

....

....

....

....

....

DIARY DATES: ....

....

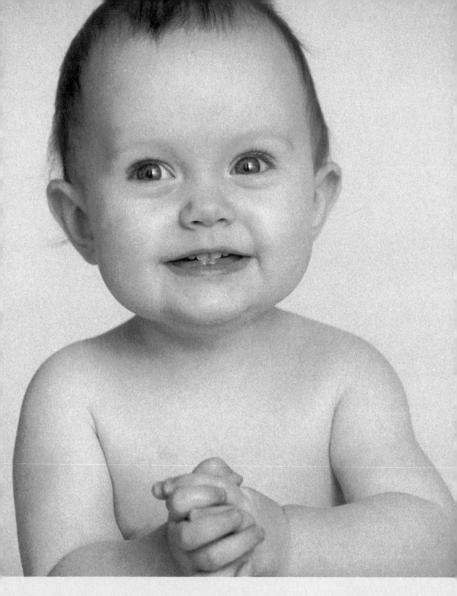

18 weeks and 1 day

day 127

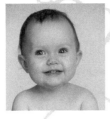

Did You Know?

It has been reported that sums of up to $75,000 have been offered for the ova of top models. However, there's no guarantee whatsoever that these eggs will produce a beautiful child. The fact is the characteristics of a child develop from a combination of both parents' genes, and one can never predict how that combination will unfold.

Thoughts and Feelings...

....

....

....

....

....

....

....

....

....

reminder

If you already have a child who is partly thrilled at the prospect of a new sibling and partly fearful, try to spend some quality time each day with them. Your life will get busier as your due date approaches and they may begin to feel left out.

DIARY DATES: ....

....

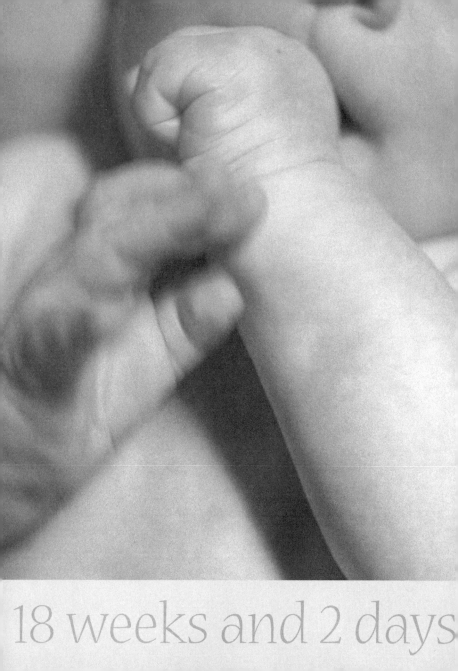

18 weeks and 2 days

day 128

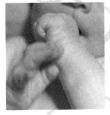

Giving Birth

If your due date has come and gone and you are beginning to feel slightly desperate, you may consider trying out one of those tried-and-tested, word-of-mouth ways to bring on labor—from spicy food to sex. Some of them are harmless—but some could be potentially dangerous. Check them out with your care provider; they won't laugh and they may even have a tip or two of their own.

Thoughts and Feelings...

....
....
....
....
....
....
....
....
....

tip · tip

IF YOU ARE OVERDUE AND FEEL LIKE YOU WANT TO SCREAM EVERY TIME SOMEONE ASKS THE OBVIOUS: "NO BABY YET?" LEAVE THE PHONE CALLS TO YOUR PARTNER. YOUR TEMPER COULD BE ON A SHORT FUSE, SO STAY CLEAR OF PEOPLE YOU FIND IRRITATING.

DIARY DATES: ....

....

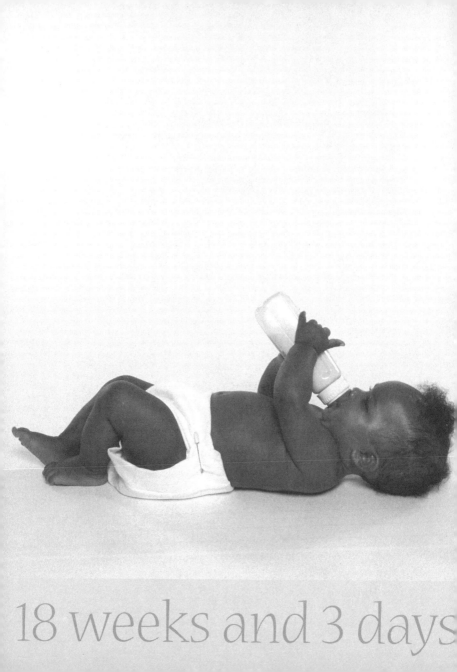

18 weeks and 3 days

day 129

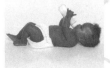

Health and Fitness

The condition of your hair may change during pregnancy. Greasy hair may improve or it may become even greasier. Dry hair can become quite brittle. Use a mild shampoo and, with dry hair, use a conditioner after every wash, and if possible allow your hair to dry naturally.

Thoughts and Feelings...

....
....
....
....
....
....
....
....
....
....

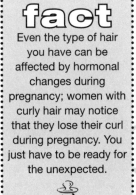

fact

Even the type of hair you have can be affected by hormonal changes during pregnancy; women with curly hair may notice that they lose their curl during pregnancy. You just have to be ready for the unexpected.

DIARY DATES: ....

....

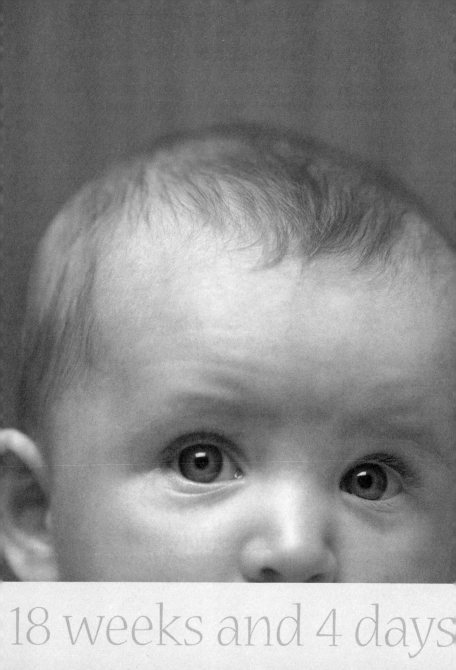
18 weeks and 4 days

day 130

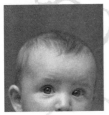

Baby's Development

The division of the nerve cells has completed and starting from this week the weight of her brain will increase by 3oz (90g) a month. The baby loses the downy hair she got about three weeks ago and is now getting coarser hair, especially on her head. The baby is now about 8¾in (22cm) long.

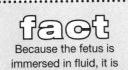

Because the fetus is immersed in fluid, it is covered in vernix caseosa, a white oily substance that acts as a protective lubricant. It stops the skin from peeling and protects against infection.

Thoughts and Feelings...

....

....

....

....

....

....

....

....

....

DIARY DATES: ....

....

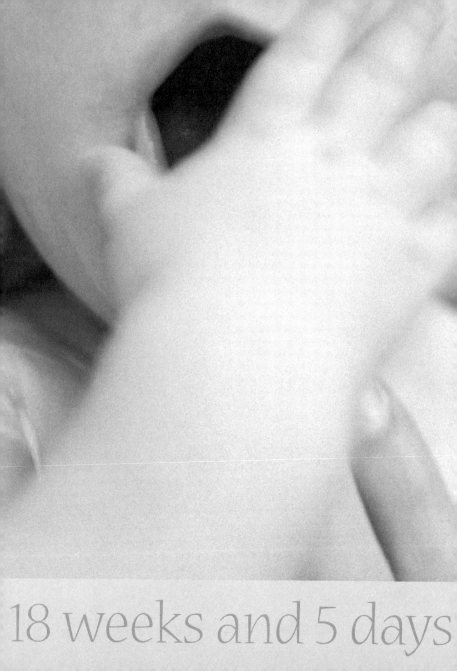

18 weeks and 5 days

day 131

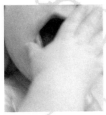

Did You Know?

One of the first signs of pregnancy is a darkening of the nipples. As your pregnancy progresses, your nipples will soften. If you have decided to breastfeed it is particularly worthwhile massaging them gently to try and make them more supple. Towards the end of your pregnancy your nipples may begin to leak, and you may need to wear breast pads to avoid staining your clothes.

"To nourish and raise children against odds is in any time, any place, more valuable than to fix bolts in cars or design nuclear weapons."

Marilyn French, author

Thoughts and Feelings…

....
....
....
....
....

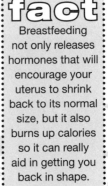

fact

Breastfeeding not only releases hormones that will encourage your uterus to shrink back to its normal size, but it also burns up calories so it can really aid in getting you back in shape.

DIARY DATES: ....

....

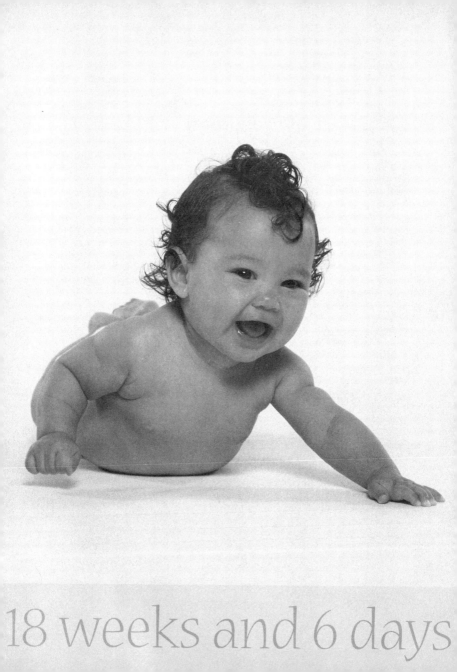

18 weeks and 6 days

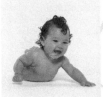

Baby Names for Girls

Jade (Spanish)
Janet (English)
Janine (English)
Jacqueline (French)
Jasmine (Arabic)
Jean (Scottish)
Jemima (Hebrew)
Jennifer (Welsh)
Jessica (Hebrew)
Jill (English)

Joanne (English)
Jocasta (Italian)
Jocelyn (English)
Jordan (English)
Josephine (Hebrew)
Joy (English)
Julia (English)
Juliet (English)
Justine (French)

Thoughts and Feelings...

....

....

....

....

....

....

....

....

tip·tip·tip·tip·tip·tip·tip·tip·tip·tip·tip·tip·tip·tip·tip·tip·tip·tip·tip·tip·tip·tip·tip·tip·tip·tip·tip·tip·tip·tip·tip·tip·tip

WERE THE
PARENTS HAVING A JOKE
OR DID THEY REALLY NOT SEE
THE OBVIOUS: WINDSOR CASTLE,
JORDAN RIVER, MINERAL WATERS, AND
GROANER DIGGER ARE JUST SOME OF THE
EXTRAORDINARY NAMES THAT HAVE BEEN
HANDED OUT.

DIARY DATES: ....

....

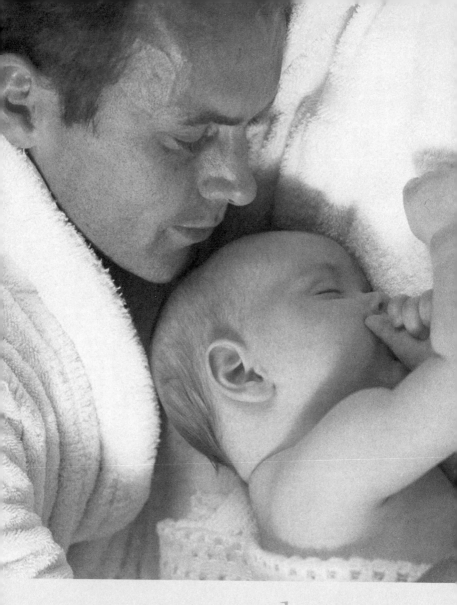

19 weeks

day 133

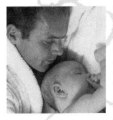

Your Pregnancy

By now you will almost certainly have felt the first movements of your baby—this is known as quickening. You are most likely to notice these when you are having a rest. When you are on the move you tend to rock the little one to sleep—when you settle down for some quiet time is when the gymnastics start. It may be a little while yet before your partner is able to feel the baby.

Thoughts and Feelings...

....
....
....
....
....
....
....
....

remember

You may be picking up all sorts of weird feelings from your tummy, so it may be a few days before you realize that the flutters you put down to gas are actually your baby moving around.

DIARY DATES: *Ask your care provider about a possible detailed ultrasound scan*

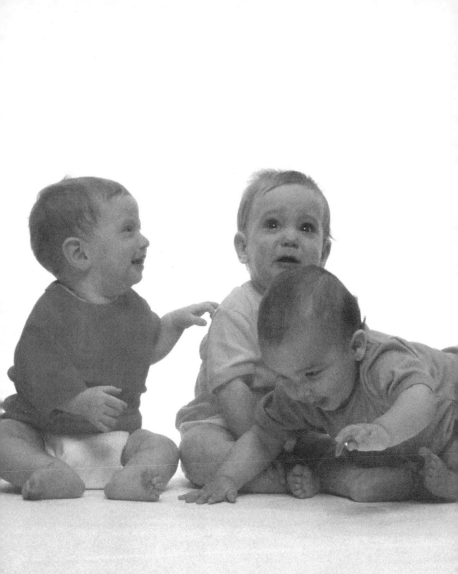

19 weeks and 1 day

day 134

Did You Know?

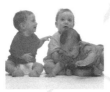

Genes are a multitude of minute little balls in which genetic material, such as eye and hair color or medical conditions, is stored. Dominant genes are genes that determine which genetic characteristics are given to the next generation; recessive genes are weak genes that are present, but which do not necessarily pass on the genetic factors.

Thoughts and Feelings...

....

....

....

....

....

....

....

....

....

fact

Genetic counsellors are trained to help you and your partner reach informed decisions about the tests available during pregnancy. They should not try to influence you to take them or tell you how you must react to the results.

DIARY DATES: ....

....

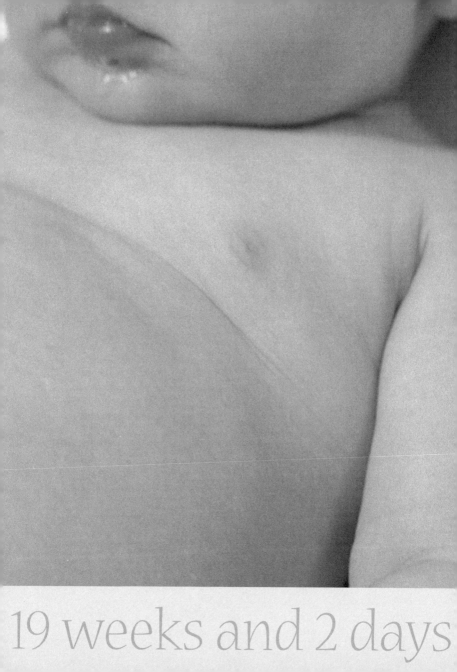

19 weeks and 2 days

19 weeks and 2 days

day 135

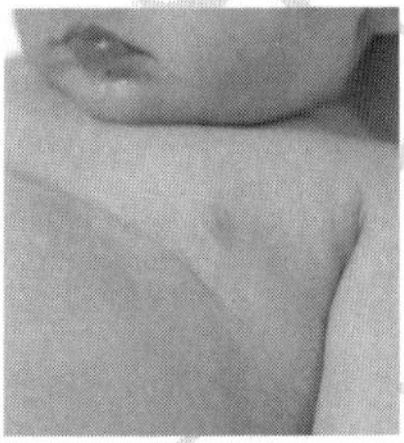

Giving Birth

A dilation contraction is when the uterus (or womb) muscle contracts, at regular intervals, causing the cervix to weaken and eventually open. The more the dilation progresses, the heavier these contractions become. The dilation contractions continue until you have dilated approximately 4in (10cm) and the baby leaves the womb via the cervix. Contractions may seem to be never ending, and learning to let go and relax between them can be vital in lasting the long haul to delivery.

fact

A fetal monitor will allow you to see your contractions as they happen. More importantly, it will also allow you to realize when a contraction is finally coming to a conclusion.

Thoughts and Feelings...

Diary Dates:

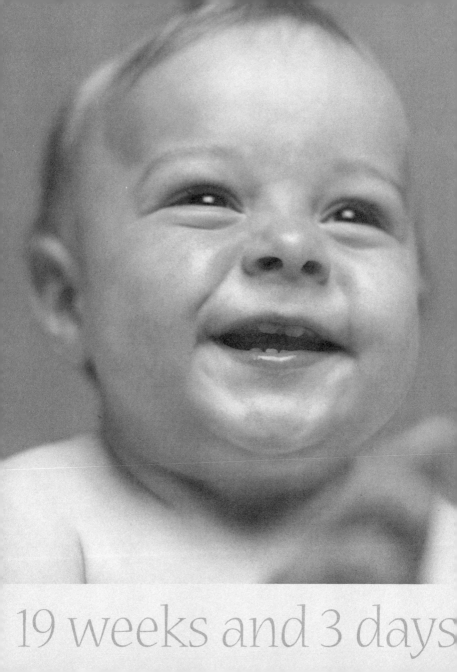

19 weeks and 3 days

day 136

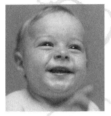

Health and Fitness

During pregnancy your teeth are extra sensitive to decay, possibly leading to cavities; your saliva contains more acids and this affects the dental enamel. In addition, weakened tissue that has an increased saturation with blood leads to more bleeding of the gums. Your dental hygiene routine needs to be attended to even more carefully. Choose a soft toothbrush and rinse several times with lukewarm, salty water or chamomile tea.

Thoughts and Feelings...

....

....

....

....

....

....

....

....

reminder

Make an appointment with the hygienist and with your dentist as well— although you will need to avoid X-rays during pregnancy. Try to see your dentist in the first few months after your baby has arrived.

DIARY DATES ....

....

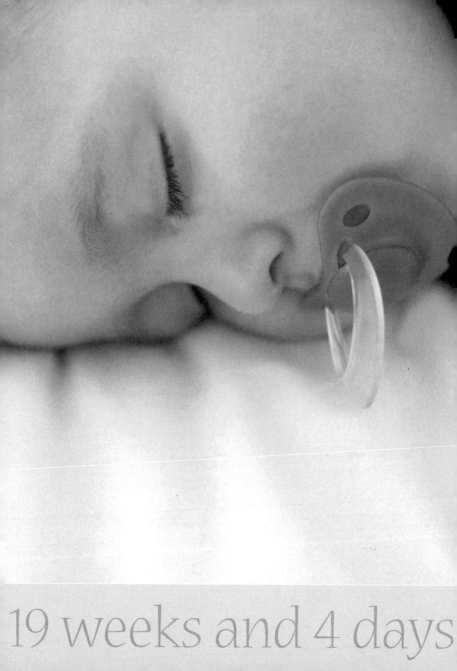

19 weeks and 4 days

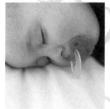

Baby's Development

The baby's hearing is now starting to work. That means that he will be startled by loud noises. The baby is moving about 200 times a day, although you certainly won't be conscious of all of them, and is roughly 10in (25cm) in length: half the length of a full-term baby. His hands can open and close freely—he has even developed his own unique fingerprints.

Thoughts and Feelings...

....

....

....

....

....

....

....

....

....

WARNING

SOME CLINICAL STUDIES HAVE FOUND A LINK BETWEEN FREQUENT EXPOSURE TO LOUD NOISES AND HIGH-FREQUENCY HEARING LOSS IN NEWBORNS. AVOID HIGH-VOLUME EVENTS, SUCH AS CONCERTS AND CLUBS, AND CHECK WITH YOUR DOCTOR ON THE RISKS OF WORKING IN A NOISY ENVIRONMENT.

DIARY DATES: ....

....

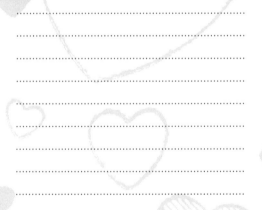

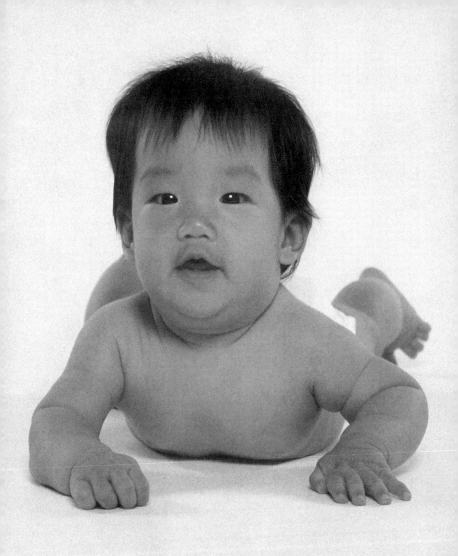

19 weeks and 5 days

day 138

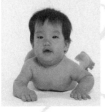

Did You Know?

Some newborns take to breastfeeding like a duck to water; others need more encouragement. Don't lose heart, as both you and the baby are new to this and with patience you will both become masters. You need to find a comfortable position for both you and the baby, then the most important thing is to make sure the baby 'latches' onto your nipple correctly.

"Children have never been very good at listening to their elders, but they have never failed to imitate them."

James Baldwin, American author (1924–1987)

Thoughts and Feelings…

....

....

....

....

....

....

....

tip · tip

A PROPER LATCH MEANS THE BABY TAKES THE WHOLE NIPPLE AND MOST OF THE AREOLA INTO HER MOUTH WITH HER NOSE VIRTUALLY ON YOUR BREAST. IT REALLY SHOULDN'T HURT. YOU WILL SEE AND HEAR YOUR BABY SWALLOWING.

DIARY DATES: ....

....

19 weeks and 6 days

day 139

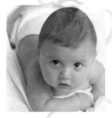

Baby Names for Boys

Jacob (Hebrew)   Jeremy (Hebrew)
James (English)   Jesse (Hebrew)
Jason (Hebrew)   John (Hebrew)
Jay (Latin)   Jonah (Hebrew)
Jeffrey (German)   Jonathan (Hebrew)

Thoughts and Feelings...

....
....
....
....
....
....
....
....
....
....
....

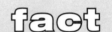
fact

The 1960s was probably
the first decade to usher
in the popularity of
unusual and even unique
names based on the
natural world.

DIARY DATES: ....
....

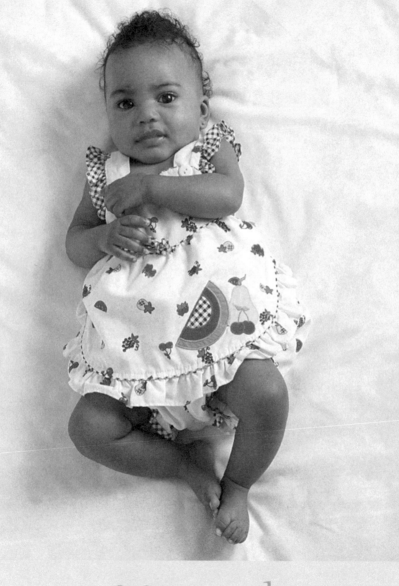

20 weeks

20 weeks

140 days to go…

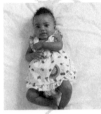

Your Pregnancy

Congratulations! Today you've put precisely half of your pregnancy behind you. That means that we're now going to count down instead of up: a countdown to your calculated due date! Your uterus and you are expanding quite rapidly now. Your navel may be pushed out or at least flattened, and as the uterus starts to push against your stomach, heartburn will become an increasing problem.

Question

How do I avoid heartburn?

· *Reduce stomach acid by drinking water between meals*

· *Eat small amounts more frequently*

· *Avoid fatty and greasy food*

· *Don't eat just before lying down to rest*

· *Use extra pillows to sleep*

Thoughts and Feelings…

....

....

....

....

....

....

....

....

....

DIARY DATES: ....

....

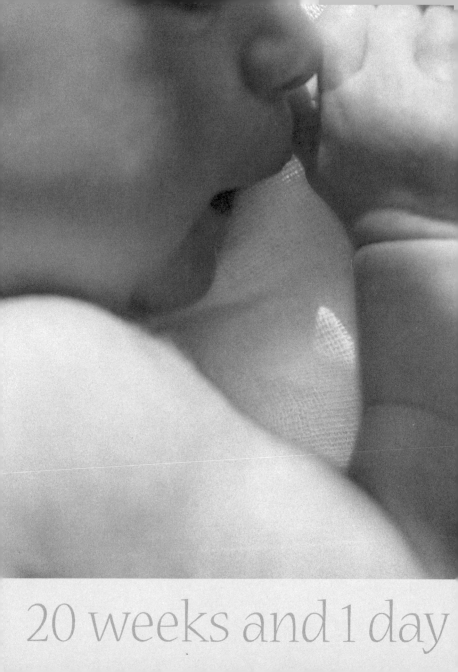

20 weeks and 1 day

139 days to go…

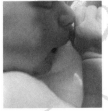

Did You Know?

It is not entirely clear why a woman who is 36 years of age or older has an increased risk of having a child with a disorder such as Down Syndrome. One theory is that because ova are already formed in a woman before she is born, some ova are busy dividing cells for dozens of years, which may result in a higher chance of disorders occurring.

Thoughts and Feelings…

....

....

....

....

....

....

....

....

....

WARNING

OLDER WOMEN ARE MORE LIKELY TO GO INTO LABOR BEFORE THEIR DUE DATE AND DELIVER PRETERM BABIES. THIS IS ONE OF THE REASONS OLDER WOMEN ARE USUALLY MONITORED MORE CAREFULLY DURING THEIR PREGNANCY.

DIARY DATES: ....

....

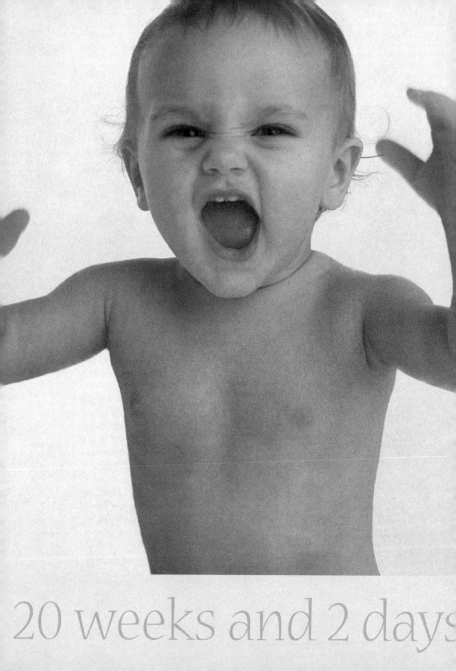

20 weeks and 2 days

138 days to go...

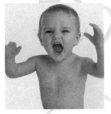

Giving Birth

During dilation the midwife will do a physical examination from time to time to feel how far the cervix has opened. The midwife inserts two fingers in the vagina and feels how flaccid the cervix is, how the membranes are doing, how deep the head is, what position the head is in, and how many inches (centimeters) you are dilated. In the (usually) long hours of dilation many women are eager to hear how far the dilation has progressed.

Thoughts and Feelings...

....
....
....
....
....
....
....
....
....

remember

You may be worrying about the physical exposure involved in childbirth; in all likelihood you won't care who sees what when the time comes as all your attention will be focused on delivering your child safely.

DIARY DATES: ....
....

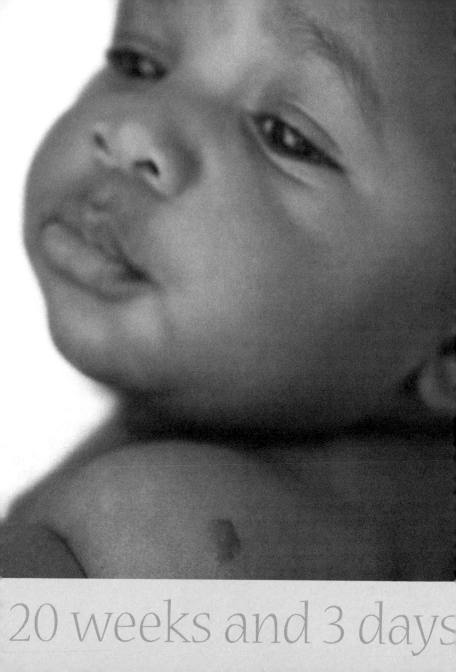

20 weeks and 3 days

137 days to go...

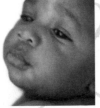

Health and Fitness

Sleeping on your left side is best for you and baby during pregnancy: the liver is positioned on the right, and lying down places your, increasingly heavy, uterus right on top of it. Sleeping on the left side will allow a free blood flow exchange with the fetus. Don't worry if you wake up on the right side, no harm will be done—simply shift back to your left side again.

Thoughts and Feelings...

....

....

....

....

....

....

....

....

....

....

fact

Water aids the exchange of nutrients between the mother and fetus. Drink three to five 8oz glasses of water over the course of the day. Caffeine causes dehydration, so drink coffee, tea, and other drinks containing caffeine in moderation.

DIARY DATES: ....

....

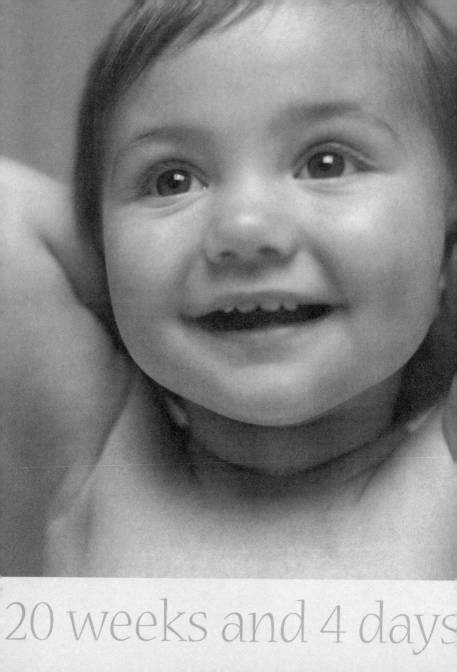

20 weeks and 4 days

136 days to go…

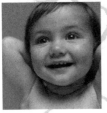

Baby's Development

Your baby is halfway through her development now. Measuring roughly 27cm (10¾in) and weighing around 13oz (365g) she is growing rapidly and making herself felt as you rapidly expand to house her. Your stomach may feel particularly dry and itchy as it changes shape, try rubbing on calamine lotion or massaging with a soothing moisturizing lotion at least once a day.

Thoughts and Feelings…

....
....
....
....
....
....
....
....
....
....

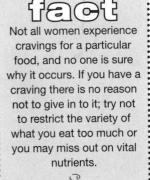

fact

Not all women experience cravings for a particular food, and no one is sure why it occurs. If you have a craving there is no reason not to give in to it; try not to restrict the variety of what you eat too much or you may miss out on vital nutrients.

DIARY DATES: ....
....

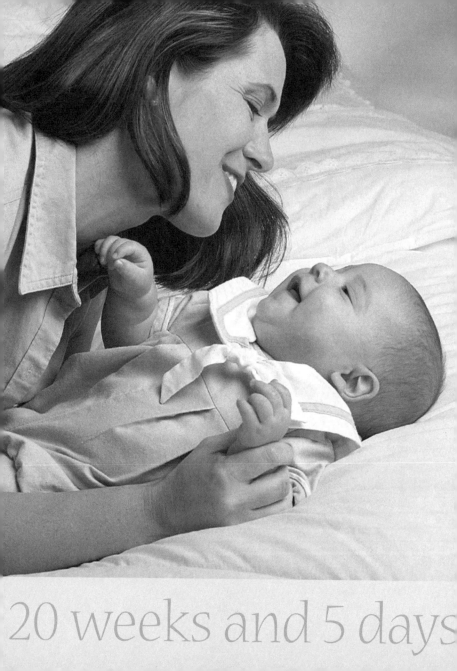

20 weeks and 5 days

135 days to go...

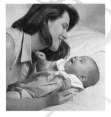

Did You Know?

You may experience restless leg syndrome (RLS) particularly in the later stages of pregnancy. Doctors are undecided on what causes this unpleasant condition that causes pain or odd sensations in the legs that can only be relieved by movement. It may be nerve compression or a deficiency of folate and/or iron. It often comes on in bed or while sitting. Talk to your care provider about treatment options.

"Your children need your presence more than your presents."

Jesse Jackson, civil rights leader

Thoughts and Feelings...

....
....
....
....
....
....
....

tip · tip ·

MANY THINGS WILL START TO CONSPIRE TO ROB YOU OF SLEEP, WHICH MAY SEEM PRECIOUS AS YOUR BODY WORKS HARD TO SUPPORT THE BABY. MAKE SURE YOU GO TO THE TOILET LAST THING AND, IF YOUR BREASTS ARE FEELING PARTICULARLY TENDER, YOU MAY FIND IT HELPFUL TO SLEEP IN A WELL-FITTING BRA.

DIARY DATES: ....
....

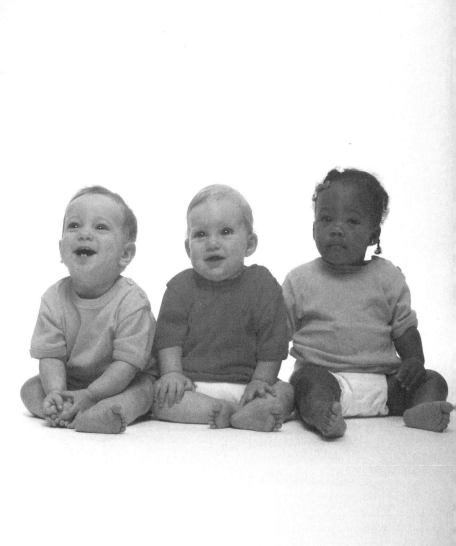

20 weeks and 6 days

134 days to go...

Baby Names for Girls

Kerry (Irish)
Kim (English)
Kimberly (English)
Kira (Bulgarian)
Kirsten (Scandinavian)

Kristen (English)
Kyle (Scottish)
Kylie (Australian Aboriginal)
Kyrie (Irish)

Thoughts and Feelings...

....
....
....
....
....
....
....
....
....
....
....

tip · tip

IN THIS AGE OF EQUALITY, SOME PARENTS MAY DECIDE TO GIVE THEIR BABY GIRL A NAME THAT COULD WORK EQUALLY WELL FOR A BABY BOY. JUST REMEMBER THIS: AS THEY GROW UP, THESE WOMEN WILL FREQUENTLY BE WRITING THEIR NAMES ON LETTERS, APPLICATIONS ETC., WHERE OTHERS WILL HAVE TO GUESS AS TO THEIR GENDER.

DIARY DATES: ....
....

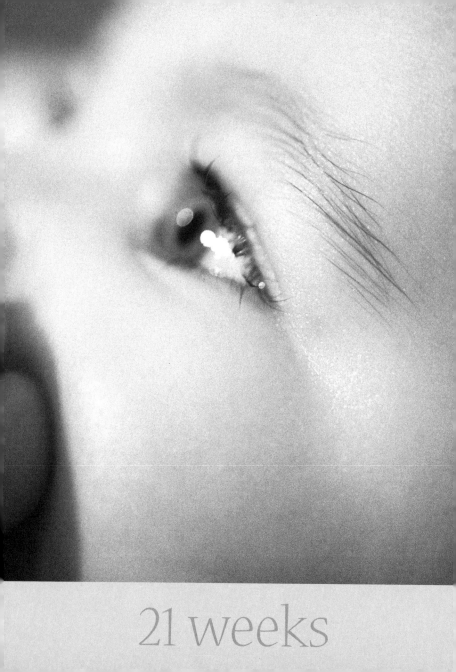

21 weeks

21 weeks

133 days to go...

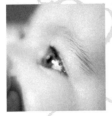

Your Pregnancy

From this point on it's important to pay attention to your posture. The hormones responsible for loosening your pelvic ligaments ready for delivery will soften other joints as well, such as your lower back ligaments and disks. Combined with the extra weight you are carrying this can lead to pain and even strains. Make sure you're wearing comfortable clothes and avoid high heels.

Thoughts and Feelings...

....

....

....

....

....

....

....

....

....

WARNING

YOU MAY ALSO EXPERIENCE ROUND LIGAMENT PAIN — THIS IS LOCATED IN YOUR LOWER ABDOMEN, INNER THIGHS AND HIPS AND IS CAUSED BY THE INCREASING WEIGHT OF YOUR UTERUS. PELVIC EXERCISES WILL KEEP THE MUSCLES IN THIS AREA TONED.

DIARY DATES: ....

....

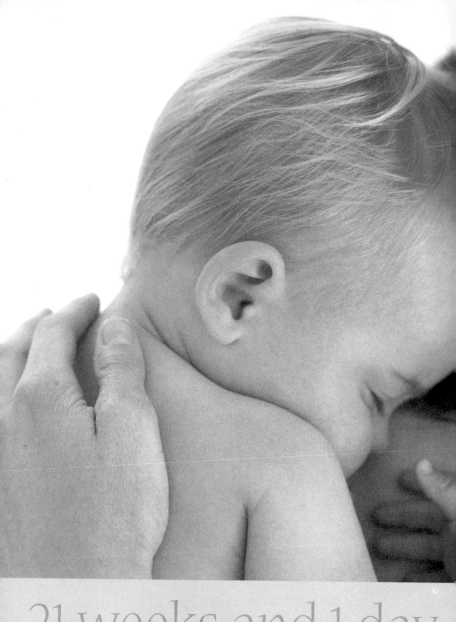

21 weeks and 1 day

21 weeks and 1 day

132 days to go...

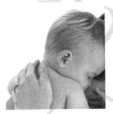

Did You Know?

Particularly towards the end of pregnancy a hot footbath can be a real pick-me-up: after all, your feet are doing a lot of extra work. You can put all kinds of things in the water to freshen up your feet: special oils, an effervescent ball or a special teabag. Explore your local body and beauty shop for some treats. Herbs like peppermint and thyme take care of and freshen up the feet.

WARNING

NOT ONLY CAN FEET SWELL OUTWARDS DURING PREGNANCY, THEY CAN ALSO EXPAND SO THAT YOU LITERALLY INCREASE A SHOE SIZE OR MORE. HAVE YOUR FEET MEASURED AND INVEST IN A REALLY COMFORTABLE PAIR OF NEW SHOES IF YOU NEED TO.

Thoughts and Feelings...

....
....
....
....
....
....
....
....
....

DIARY DATES: ....
....

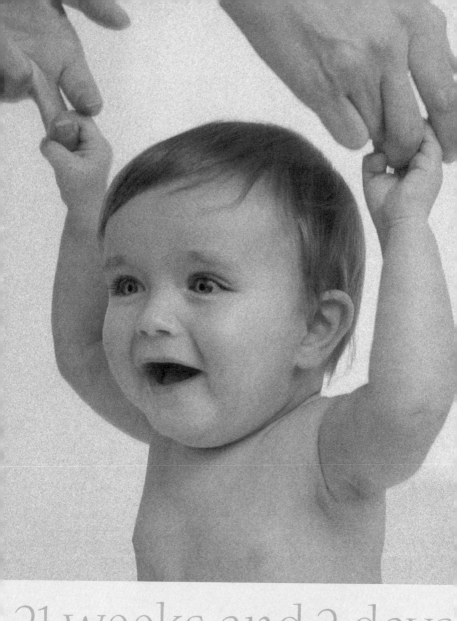

21 weeks and 2 days

131 days to go...

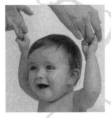

Giving Birth

Dilation of the cervix doesn't show at all on the outside. The only way to find out what is happening is for the midwife to do an internal examination. She will use sterile gloves and wipe the area around the entrance to the vagina with an antiseptic because—once your waters have broken in particular—there is always a chance of infection. For this reason internal exams will be kept to a minimum.

Thoughts and Feelings...

....

....

....

....

....

....

....

....

....

....

fact

There are many different types of pain relief available from alternative therapies such as acupuncture to quite major medical interventions such as an epidural. Only you can decide if and when you want to take pain relief, so make sure you are well informed on the options.

DIARY DATES: ....

....

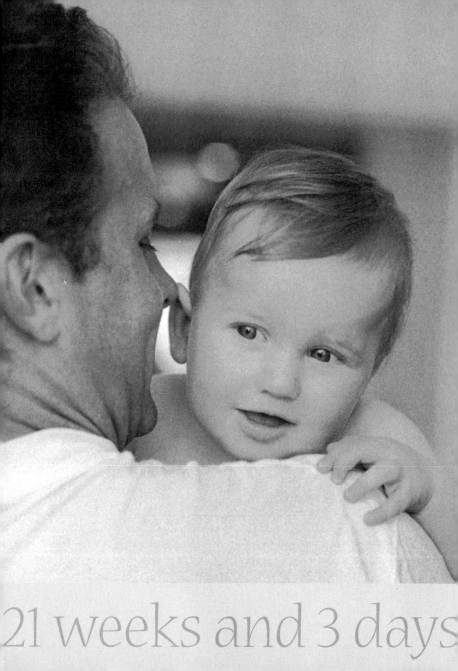

21 weeks and 3 days

130 days to go...

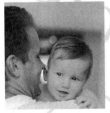

Health and Fitness

Be careful with the sun and the sun bed. During pregnancy your skin may become even more sensitive to the sun's rays. Chloasma (changes in skin pigment) may cause a mask-like darkening or lightening of the facial skin and moles are prone to darkening. Wear a high-factor sunscreen (factor 30 or above) and spend as much time

Thoughts and Feelings...

....
....
....
....
....
....
....
....
....
....

WARNING

DON'T LIE ON YOUR BACK TO SLEEP DURING PREGNANCY. THE VEIN CARRYING BLOOD FROM YOUR FEET AND LEGS TO YOUR HEART MAY GET BLOCKED CAUSING A DROP IN BLOOD PRESSURE. YOUR ONLY OPTION NOW IS YOUR LEFT SIDE.

DIARY DATES: ....

....

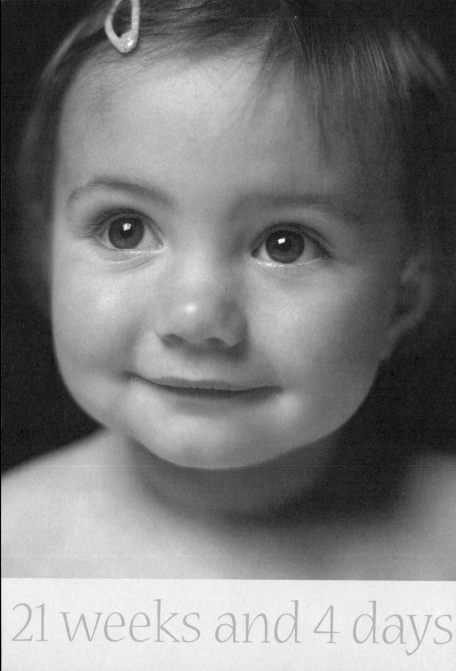

21 weeks and 4 days

129 days to go…

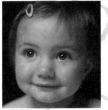

Baby's Development

The genitals of a girl are developing quickly now. Millions of eggs have already been produced in the ovaries; however, these start to reduce immediately and by the time of the birth will already be down to one to two million. They will continue decreasing until puberty. The baby is about 11¼in (28.5cm) long and her tiny fingers already have nails.

Thoughts and Feelings…

....

....

....

....

....

....

....

....

....

....

....

tip · tip ·

IF YOUR BABY'S ACROBATICS ARE KEEPING YOU AWAKE AT NIGHT, TRY STROKING YOUR STOMACH AND TALKING TO THE BABY SOFTLY. YOUR BABY WILL BE SOOTHED BY THE SOUND OF YOUR VOICE AND MAY BE ENCOURAGED TO LET YOU GET SOME MORE SLEEP!

DIARY DATES: ....

....

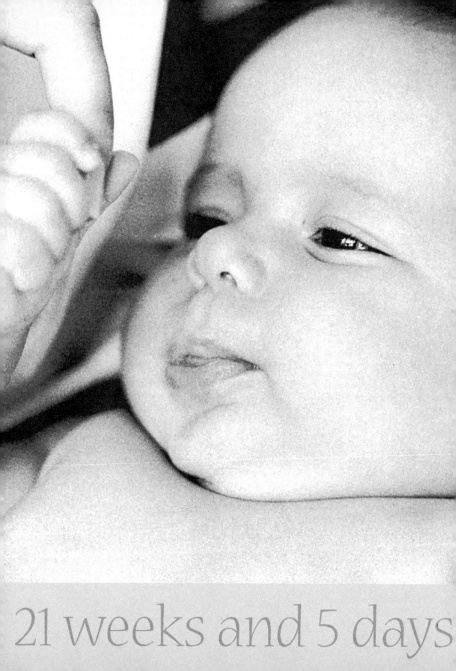

21 weeks and 5 days

128 days to go...

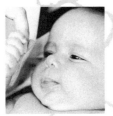

"I don't know if it's got anything to do with my age but I'm always tired. I think anyone with three children knows that it's always going to be two versus three. You don't have the energy left to save the world anymore because you're always needed at home. If I go out for an evening, at home it's always 'Where are you going? You're not allowed to!' But it isn't so bad that I need to call help in. Imagine that!"

Susan Sarandon, actress, had her third child at age 45

(taken from *Beau Monde*)

Thoughts and Feelings...

....

....

....

....

....

....

....

fact

The trend in Western cultures is for small families. In some Mediterranean countries such as Italy, where birth rates have fallen dramatically, but the average number of children in the UK is now just one.

DIARY DATES: ....

....

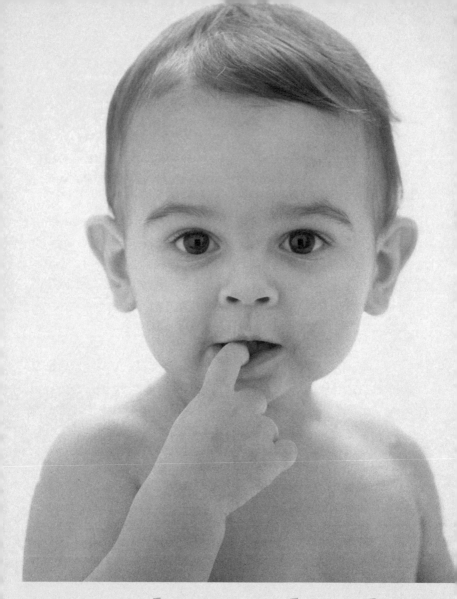

21 weeks and 6 days

127 days to go...

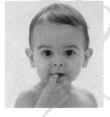

Baby Names for Boys

Karl (German)
Keith (Scottish)
Kelly (Irish)
Kelvin (African American)
Kenneth (Irish)

Kerry (Irish)
Kevin (Irish)
Kiefer (German)
Kieran (Irish)
Kyle (Scottish)

Thoughts and Feelings...

....
....
....
....
....
....
....
....
....
....
....

DIARY DATES: ....
....

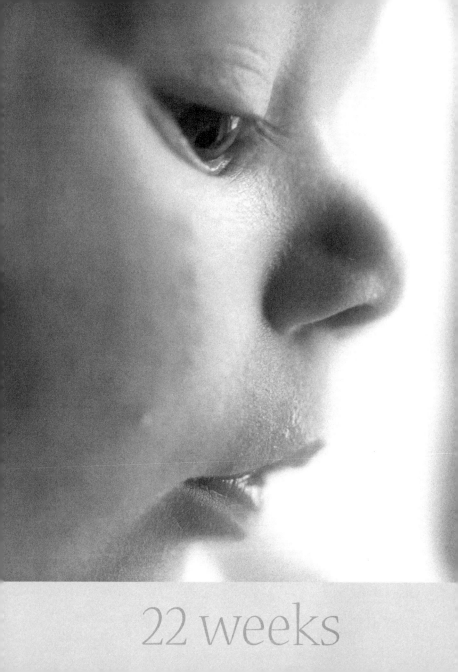

22 weeks

126 days to go...

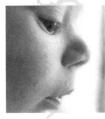

Your Pregnancy

The changes in your body are becoming abundantly clear: larger breasts, your stomach is growing rapidly, and your waistline has just about disappeared. If you are genetically predisposed to them you will develop stretch marks, and there is nothing you can do to stop them. These white, red, or purple fine lines may develop on your stomach, breasts, legs, or any other part of your expanding body.

Thoughts and Feelings...

....
....
....
....
....
....
....
....
....

DIARY DATES: ....
....

Q&A
Do stretch marks stay forever?

Stretch marks should fade to very fine white lines soon after pregnancy. If you are extremely self-conscious about them, studies have shown that Retin A and laser treatment can help; talk to your doctor about your options.

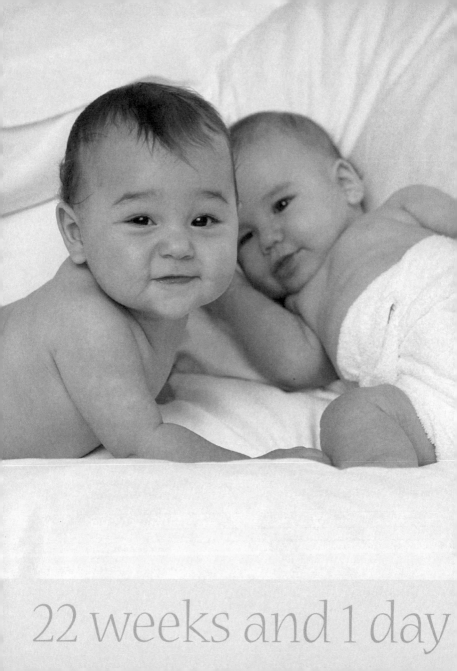

22 weeks and 1 day

125 days to go...

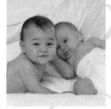

Did You Know?

If you are still undecided about whether or not to breastfeed, childbirth classes can offer valuable information about the pros and cons of breast and bottle feeding. If you have difficulty breastfeeding successfully to begin with you may find the nurses at the hospital where you delivered helpful and if they have a lactation specialist on staff you may be able to talk to them or make an appointment to see them.

Thoughts and Feelings...

....

....

....

....

....

....

....

....

....

remember

The La Leche League is available to help and support women who wish to breastfeed. They will be able to put you in touch with other women who can offer emotional support as well as practical guidance and advice.

DIARY DATES: ....

....

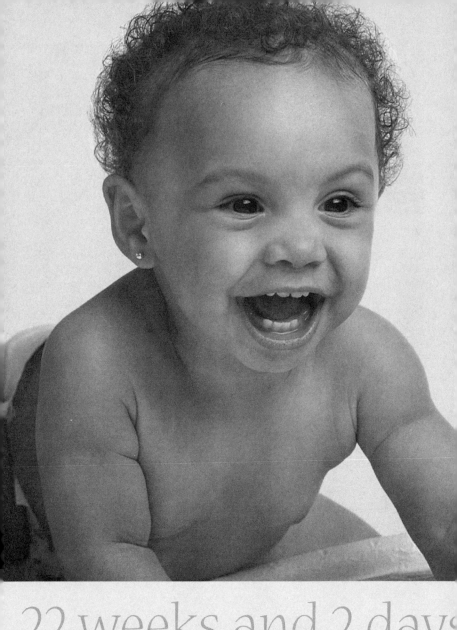

22 weeks and 2 days

124 days to go...

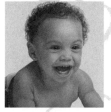

Giving Birth

If you approach labor with a negative mindset, convinced it is going to be a painful and traumatic experience, you may increase the chances of an unnecessarily painful delivery! Try to embark on this journey with an open mind, reacting to the experience as it actually happens to you. If you find the pain unbearable, then that is the time to ask for some help.

Thoughts and Feelings...

....

....

....

....

....

....

....

....

fact

Certain procedures for relieving pain—in particular an epidural—can only be employed at certain points of the labor process, not at the very end. Be sure to discuss as early as possible with your doctor, nurse, or midwife what pain-relief options you are considering.

DIARY DATES: ....

....

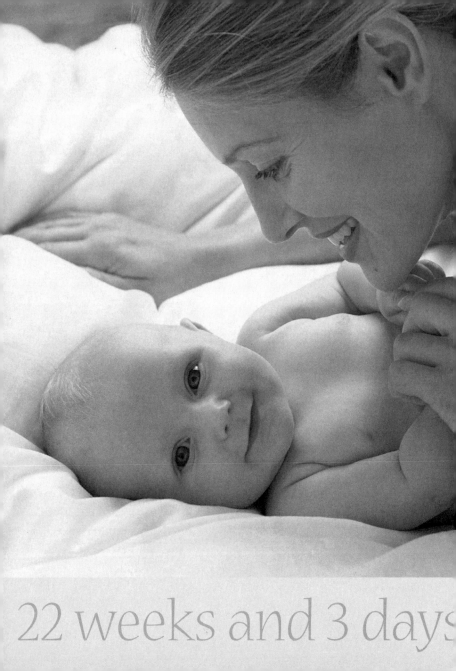

22 weeks and 3 days

123 days to go...

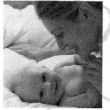

Health and Fitness

On average, women put on between 22–30lb (10–14kg) during pregnancy. These extra kilos are roughly distributed as follows: 3–4kg 6½–8¾lb (3–4kg) for the baby; 21–28oz (600–800g) for the placenta; 2lb (1kg) for the womb; 14oz (400g) for the breasts; 2lb (1kg) for the waters (amniotic fluid); 3lb 2oz (1.5kg) of extra blood; 3lb (1.4kg) of extra body fluid; and 7¾lb (3.5kg) of extra body fat (necessary for breastfeeding).

Thoughts and Feelings...

....
....
....
....
....
....
....
....
....

tip · tip ·

IF YOU FIND YOUR LEGS ARE STARTING TO ACHE WITH THE EXTRA WEIGHT THEY HAVE TO CARRY AROUND, TRY MASSAGING THEM WITH A MOISTURIZER AFTER YOUR BATH OR SHOWER. TRY TO REST, AS MUCH AS POSSIBLE, WITH YOUR LEGS RAISED UP.

DIARY DATES: ....
....

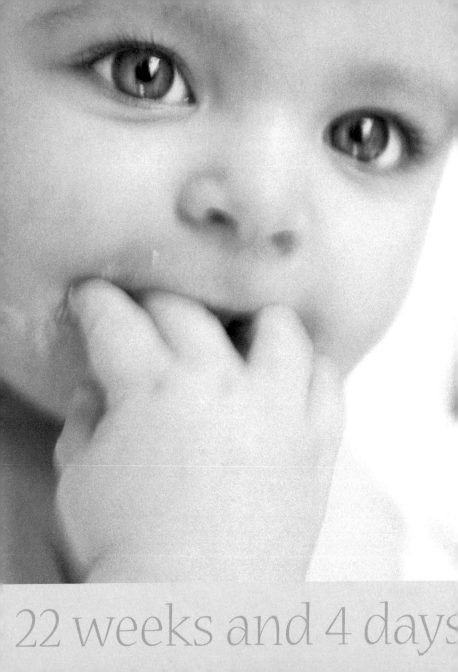

22 weeks and 4 days

122 days to go…

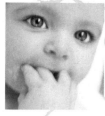

Baby's Development

You can really start to bond with your little one now, and stroking your stomach and perhaps tapping lightly may increase the chance of a reaction. The baby may cough and if you experience a rhythmic jerking from your abdomen it is likely she has hiccoughs. This is caused by drinking and/or breathing amniotic fluid, and will pass off with time. The baby is growing fast now and is measuring roughly 12in (30.5cm) long.

WARNING

AS THE BABY GETS MORE NIMBLE, YOU MAY FIND YOURSELF GETTING INCREASINGLY CLUMSY. AS YOUR CENTRE OF GRAVITY SHIFTS IT IS EASY TO BUMP INTO THINGS. TAKE PARTICULAR CARE IF YOU ARE HAVING A WINTER PREGNANCY, AS YOU COULD EASILY SLIP ON ICY PATHS.

Thoughts and Feelings…

....

....

....

....

....

....

....

....

....

DIARY DATES: ....

....

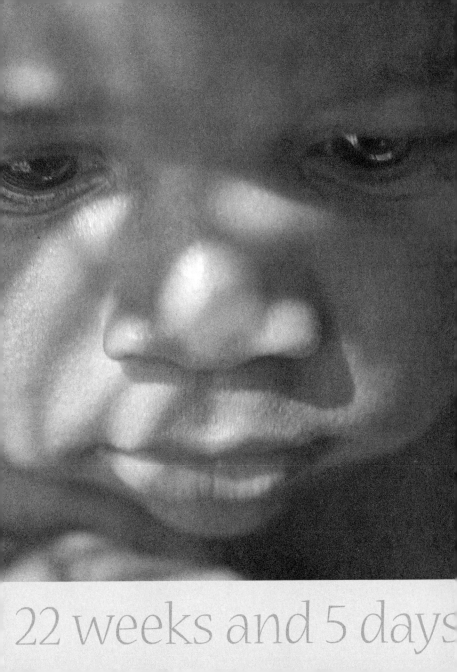
22 weeks and 5 days

121 days to go...

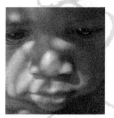

"Despite being famous we really try to make sure that we don't isolate ourselves. It's not good for us and definitely not good for our children. I just love spending time with my children, even more so because my own father was hardly ever around. I don't want to be a father like that for my children."

Tom Cruise, actor, speaking about his two adopted children

(taken from *IQ*)

Thoughts and Feelings...

....

....

....

....

....

....

....

....

reminder

Many new parents worry about their parenting skills: it isn't necessary to be the best parent in the world, actually being there for your children is the most important thing.

DIARY DATES: ....

....

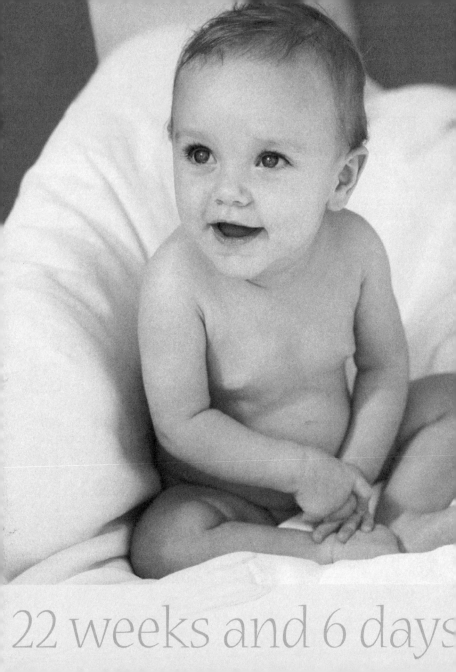

22 weeks and 6 days

120 days to go...

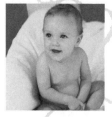

Baby Names for Girls

Lara (English)
Laura (Latin)
Linda (Spanish)
Lindsay (English)
Lisa (English)
Lorna (Scottish)

Lorraine (French)
Louise (English)
Lucy (English)
Lydia (Greek)
Lynn (English)

Thoughts and Feelings...

fact

In Kenya, children may receive several names. The first comes from the maternal side of the family and is a birth name. A month or so later, the parents or the paternal side of the family choose a more permanent name.

....
....
....
....
....
....
....
....
....
....
....

DIARY DATES: ....
....

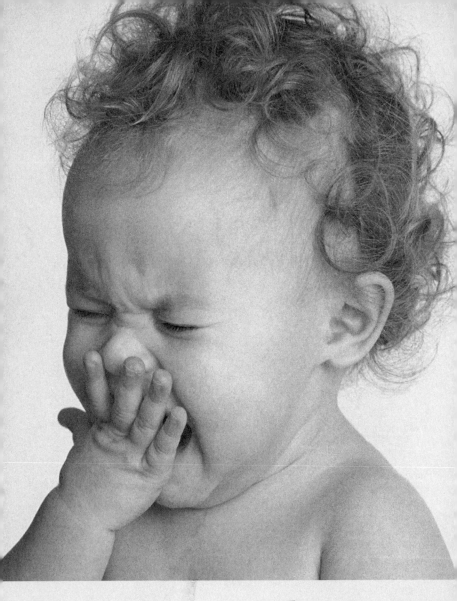

23 weeks

23 weeks

119 days to go...

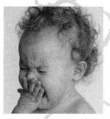

Your Pregnancy

Now you have passed the morning sickness mark and before you hit the burden of late pregnancy you may feel in the mood for some renewed sexual intimacy with your partner. After all, you don't have to worry about contraception and the challenge of finding new positions to accommodate your new shape may add extra spice to your sex life.

Thoughts and Feelings...

....

....

....

....

....

....

....

....

....

....

WARNING

ORAL SEX CAN BE A REWARDING OPTION AT THIS STAGE OF YOUR PREGNANCY. JUST MAKE SURE YOUR PARTNER DOES NOT BLOW INTO YOUR VAGINA AS THERE IS A RARE, BUT REAL, RISK OF AN AIR EMBOLISM.

DIARY DATES: ....

....

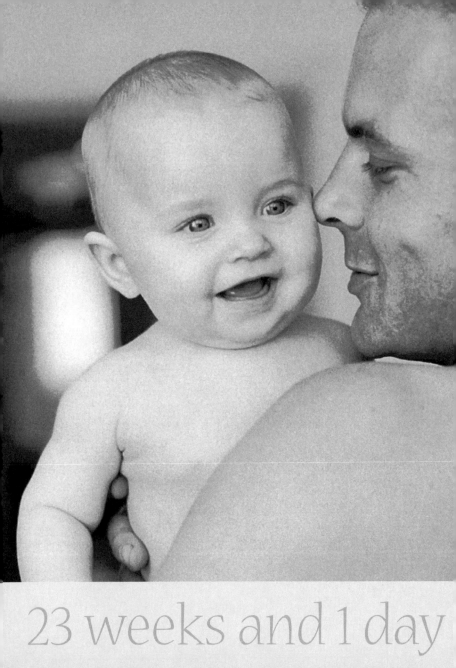

23 weeks and 1 day

118 days to go...

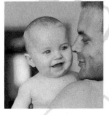

Did You Know?

Sometimes waiting for the arrival of a new baby can leave you with a feeling that you have too much to do and too little time in which to achieve it. It would be lovely to pamper yourself, but this can take up time and money. Instead, use the cash to tick some jobs off your chore list: pay someone to clean your house, paint the baby's room, or do your shopping for a few weeks.

Thoughts and Feelings...

....

....

....

....

....

....

....

....

....

tip · tip ·

IF CASH AND TIME ARE NOT TOO PRESSING, TREAT YOURSELF TO A DAY AT A HEALTH SPA OR AN AFTERNOON MATINEE. THESE ARE THINGS YOU MAY LOOK BACK ON FONDLY WHEN YOUR DAYS ARE FILLED WITH CARING FOR A NEW BABY.

DIARY DATES: ....

....

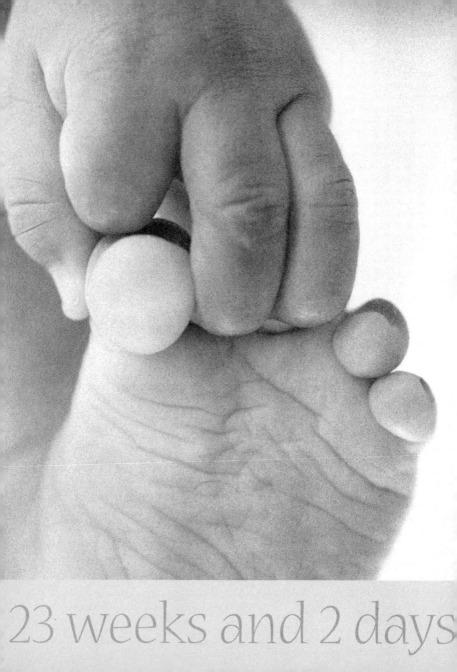

23 weeks and 2 days

117 days to go…

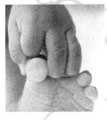

Giving Birth

The pushing or second phase is when the child is pushed out of the womb by the contractions and by the mother pushing as well. The baby makes its way through the birth canal to the outside world. During dilation the birth canal becomes increasingly soft and flaccid; the resistance of the tissue is reduced and as a result it

Thoughts and Feelings…

....

....

....

....

....

....

....

....

....

....

tip · tip ·

THE OPTIMUM TIME FOR PUSHING IS AT THE PEAK OF A CONTRACTION. CONCENTRATE ALL YOUR EFFORTS ON PUSHING EFFECTIVELY: DON'T WORRY ABOUT ANY WEIRD GRUNTS AND MOANING THAT MAY ACCOMPANY THIS—THE PROFESSIONALS ATTENDING YOUR BIRTH WILL MOST CERTAINLY HAVE HEARD IT ALL BEFORE.

DIARY DATES: ....

....

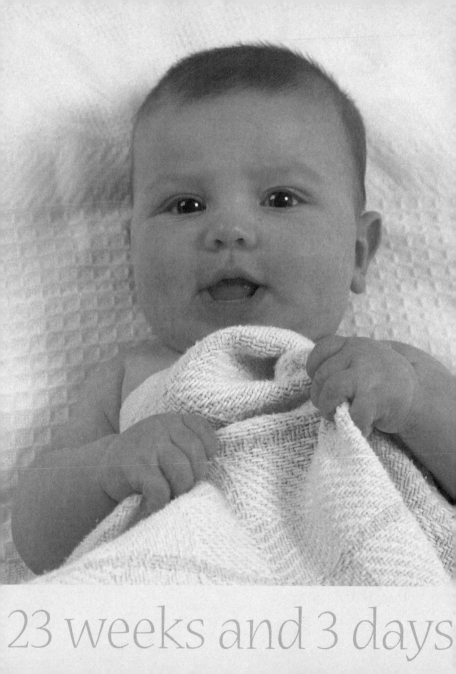

23 weeks and 3 days

23 weeks and 3 days

116 days to go...

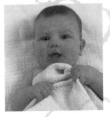

Health and Fitness

Swimming is an excellent sport to take up during pregnancy. It is good for the muscles and stamina as well as being relaxing—and can be done throughout the pregnancy. The water makes you weightless, which can be an extremely pleasant sensation, particularly towards the end of the pregnancy. Invest in a good maternity swimsuit if you plan to swim regularly, or wear an old bikini with a T-shirt over the top.

Thoughts and Feelings...

....

....

....

....

....

....

....

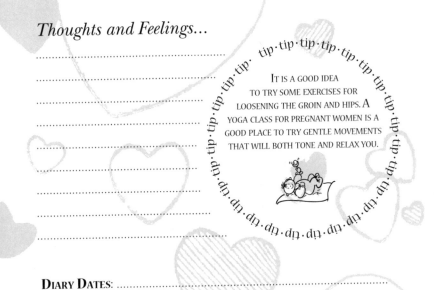

tip·tip·tip·tip·tip·tip·tip·tip·tip·tip·tip·tip·tip·tip·tip·tip·tip·tip·tip·tip·tip·tip

IT IS A GOOD IDEA TO TRY SOME EXERCISES FOR LOOSENING THE GROIN AND HIPS. A YOGA CLASS FOR PREGNANT WOMEN IS A GOOD PLACE TO TRY GENTLE MOVEMENTS THAT WILL BOTH TONE AND RELAX YOU.

DIARY DATES: ....

....

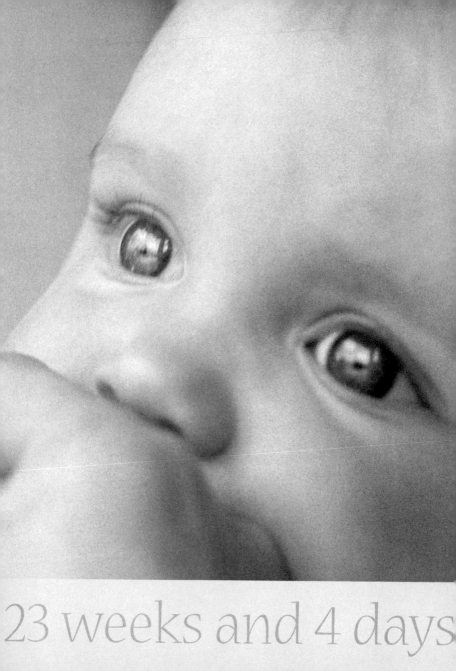

23 weeks and 4 days

115 days to go...

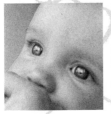

Baby's Development

The fetus now makes roughly 20 to 60 movements every 30 seconds. That varies throughout the day as the baby has periods of wakefulness and times when he prefers to sleep: and this pattern may continue after birth. Noises and movement from outside can also disturb your baby. The heartbeat can be heard easily with an ordinary stethoscope now, and baby is 312½in (32cm) long.

Thoughts and Feelings...

....

....

....

....

....

....

....

....

....

WARNING

YOU MAY OCCASIONALLY FEEL A STITCH-LIKE PAIN DOWN THE SIDE OF YOUR STOMACH. THIS IS YOUR UTERUS MUSCLE STRETCHING. TRY TO TAKE A REST AND THE PAIN SHOULD SOON GO AWAY.

DIARY DATES: ....

....

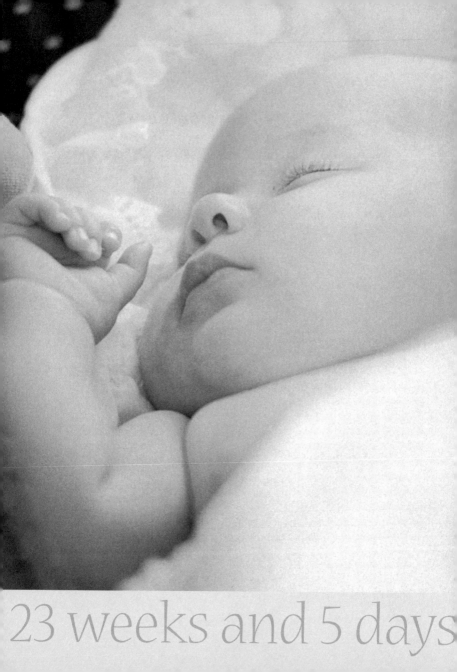

23 weeks and 5 days

114 days to go...

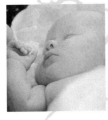

Did You Know?

A birth plan should be a guide for how you would like the delivery of your baby to go. You cannot account for everything that happens on the day and you need to accept that the midwife or doctor attending will have the well being of both you and your baby as their first priority. Medical emergencies do happen, and in this case you need to follow the advice you are given.

Thoughts and Feelings...

....

....

....

....

....

....

....

tip · tip

IF YOUR CARE PROVIDER SEEMS RESISTANT TO YOUR BIRTH PLAN, TRY TO SIT DOWN AND REALLY LISTEN TO THE ISSUES THEY RAISE. ARE THEY TRYING TO TELL YOU PART OF YOUR PLAN IS UNREALISTIC? TRY TO DECIDE ON A COMPROMISE BETWEEN BOTH OF YOU.

DIARY DATES: ....

....

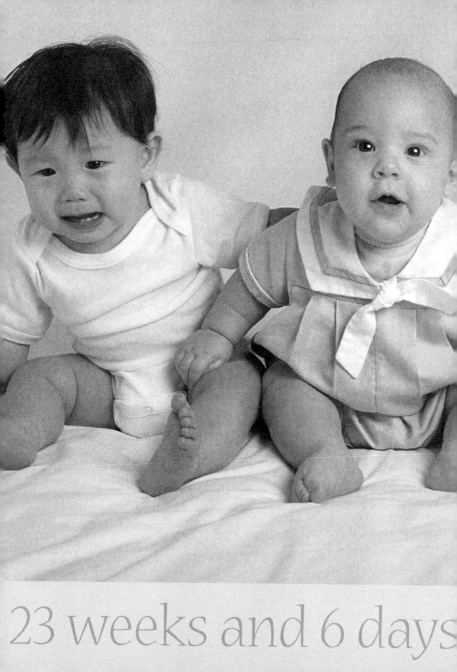

23 weeks and 6 days

113 days to go...

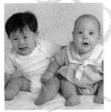

Baby Names for Boys

Larry (English)	Leslie (Scottish)
Lawrence (English)	Lester (English)
Lee (English)	Lionel (Latin)
Lennox (Scottish)	Louis (French)
Leon (Greek)	Lucas (English)
Leonard (German)	

WARNING

THERE IS NO GETTING AWAY FROM THE FACT THAT NAMES ARE EVOCATIVE. IF THEY BRING TO MIND SOMEONE WE LIKE, WE TEND TO LIKE THE NAME AND PEOPLE WITH THAT NAME. UNFORTUNATELY, IF IT REMINDS OF SOMEONE WE DISLIKE, IT MAY PREJUDICE US AGAINST EVERYONE WITH THAT NAME.

Thoughts and Feelings...

....
....
....
....
....
....
....
....
....

DIARY DATES: ....
....

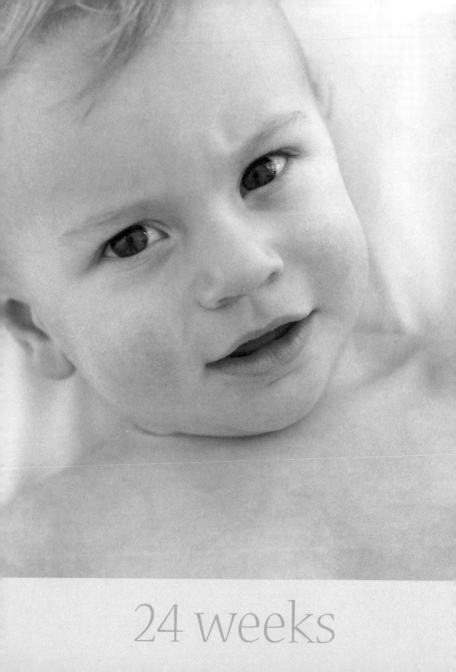

24 weeks

112 days to go...

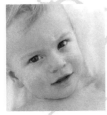

Your Pregnancy

Because of their rapidly growing belly, pregnant women often tend to start walking with a hollow back and this can result in back pain. It is very important to concentrate on good posture: not only in walking but also while sitting. Remember to use right practice if you have to pick something up from the floor—especially if this is a small toddler—and always bend from the knees, not the back.

Thoughts and Feelings...

....

....

....

....

....

....

....

....

....

WARNING

AVOID SUDDEN MOVEMENTS: WITH EVERYTHING LOOSENED BY PREGNANCY HORMONES IT IS ESPECIALLY EASY TO PULL OR STRAIN A MUSCLE. EVEN GETTING OUT OF BED CAN BE A HAZARD: ALWAYS ROLL ON TO YOUR SIDE AND USE YOUR ARMS TO HELP YOU SIT UP.

DIARY DATES: Routine check-up

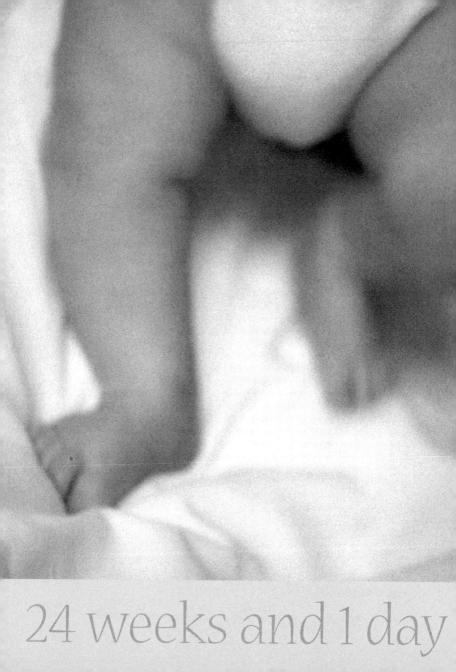

24 weeks and 1 day

111 days to go...

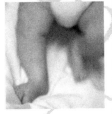

Did You Know?

During pregnancy, hormones work to weaken the ligaments to makes it easier for the child to go through the birth canal during delivery. This can cause an imbalance of the pelvis. This is called pelvic instability. Women suffering from pelvic instability often complain about constant pain in their pubic bone, tailbone, hips, and lower back and have trouble cycling, bending over, standing for a long time, and making love. Consult your doctor if you are worried that you may have this condition.

Thoughts and Feelings...

....

....

....

....

....

....

....

....

....

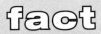

If you find you are suffering from lower back pain, a maternity support belt that fits around your back and underneath your bump may help to carry the extra weight of your belly and support your back. They are available from maternity shops and department stores.

DIARY DATES: ....

....

24 weeks and 2 days

110 days to go...

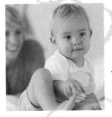

Giving Birth

The transitional phase is one of the most challenging parts of labour. It is the time just before pushing starts, and yet the cervix still has to dilate a few more centimetres to allow the child's head through. Your body may be urging you to push – but this is wasted effort and your care provider will be making sure that you don't. One sign of the transitional phase is the unpredictability of the contractions.

Thoughts and Feelings...

....
....
....
....
....
....
....
....
....
....

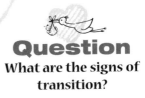

Question

What are the signs of transition?

· *Back pain*

· *Chills and sweats*

· *Sickness and even vomiting*

· *Contractions very close together or unpredictable*

· *An urge to push*

· *Rectal pressure from the baby*

DIARY DATES: ....
....

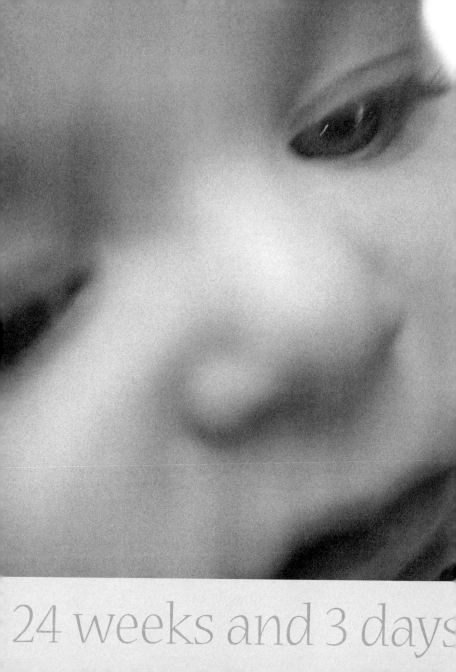

24 weeks and 3 days

109 days to go...

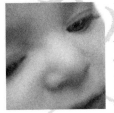

Health and Fitness

Sufficient sleep is a free and highly necessary beauty product, especially during pregnancy. Try to sleep at least eight hours a night and have small rests during the day. However, you may find that just when you need it most, sleep is hard to find. Keep your bedroom cool to cope with your raised metabolism and perhaps leave a light on to help you navigate your way to the bathroom for those inevitable nighttime calls.

Thoughts and Feelings...

....

....

....

....

....

....

....

....

tip · tip ·

IF SLEEPING ON YOUR SIDE IS GIVING YOU PAIN IN YOUR SHOULDERS AND HIPS, YOU COULD TRY SOME EXTRA PADDING ON YOUR MATTRESS, USING SOME TEXTURED FOAM. A PILLOW PLACED UNDER YOUR BUMP CAN ALSO ADD EXTRA SUPPORT.

DIARY DATES: ....

....

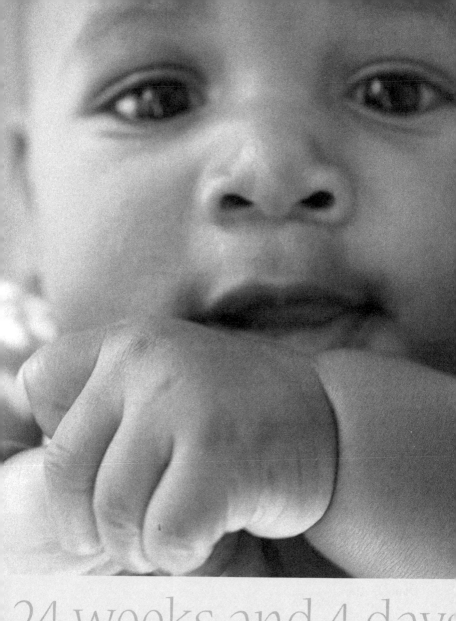

24 weeks and 4 days

108 days to go…

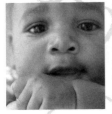

Baby's Development

Your growing baby is no longer floating around loosely in the amniotic fluid, but neither has he taken up his final position. The fetus is beginning to look more like a newborn with his head in better proportion to the rest of his body. He still looks very wrinkled, but the first bit of subcutaneous fat is now being formed. Already a boy will be a bit heavier than a girl. your baby measures roughly 12¾in (32.5cm) in length.

Thoughts and Feelings…

....
....
....
....
....
....
....
....
....

reminder

Even if you choose childbirth classes independent from the hospital where you are going to deliver, it is worth contacting them for a tour of the maternity ward. You need to know where you are going to and what to expect on the day.

DIARY DATES: ....
....

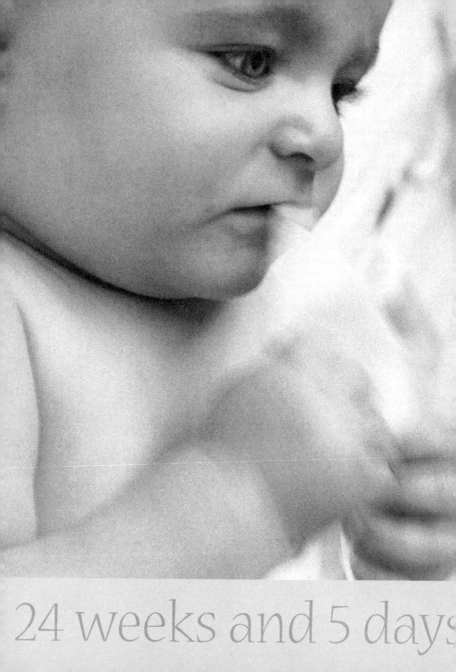

24 weeks and 5 days

107 days to go...

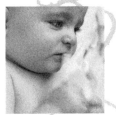

"She's the best thing that's ever happened to me. It's just amazing how much I love her. It's the first love relationship in my life that comes without any catches. She doesn't know I'm famous and hasn't the slightest idea about my life. It's unconditional love."

Madonna, singer and actress (taken from *Avant Garde*)

Thoughts and Feelings...

....

....

....

....

....

....

....

....

....

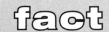

Breastfeeding or not, people do sometimes get pregnant again very shortly after giving birth. Even if sex seems unlikely, consider your contraceptive options in advance unless you would like a repeat visit to the maternity ward.

DIARY DATES: ....

....

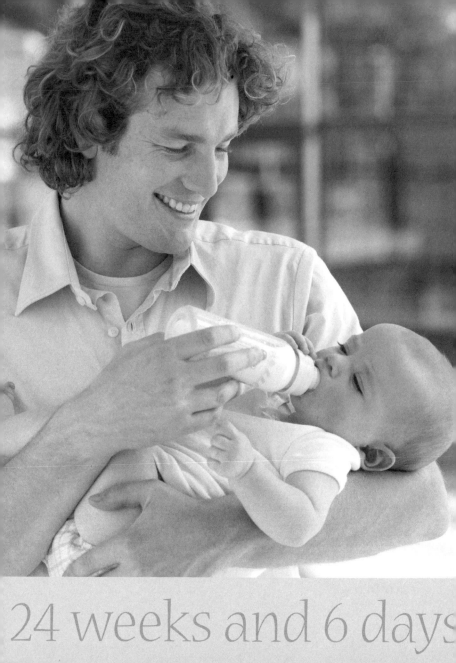

24 weeks and 6 days

106 days to go…

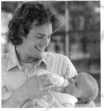

Baby Names for Girls

Madeline (French)

Marcia (Latin)

Margaret (English)

Marie (French)

Martha (English)

Mary (Hebrew)

Matilda (Old German)

Maureen (Irish)

Maxine (English)

Melanie (Greek)

Michelle (French)

Miranda (Latin)

Monica (Latin)

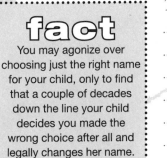

fact

You may agonize over choosing just the right name for your child, only to find that a couple of decades down the line your child decides you made the wrong choice after all and legally changes her name. Over 50,000 people a year in the United States do just that.

Thoughts and Feelings…

....

....

....

....

....

....

....

....

....

....

DIARY DATES: ....

....

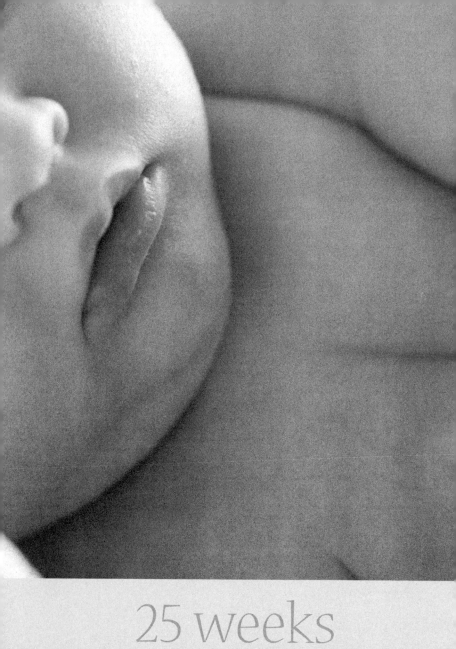

25 weeks

25 weeks

105 days to go...

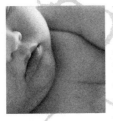

Your Pregnancy

You may be suffering from fluid retention, causing puffy and aching feet and legs. Your increased blood volume and high levels of oestrogen are mostly to blame. Plenty of rest with the feet raised will help, as will a pair of support stockings. Don't restrict your fluid intake and, although sodium should be taken in moderation, you do need slightly more during pregnancy.

Thoughts and Feelings...

....

....

....

....

....

....

....

....

....

....

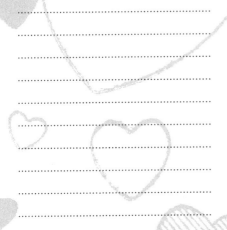

WARNING

IF YOU SUDDENLY FIND YOUR FACE AND HANDS HAVE SWOLLEN UP, CONTACT YOUR DOCTOR IMMEDIATELY AS IT COULD BE AN INDICATION OF PREECLAMPSIA OR TOXEMIA (BLOOD POISONING), BOTH OF WHICH ARE DANGEROUS CONDITIONS FOR YOU AND THE BABY.

DIARY DATES: ....

....

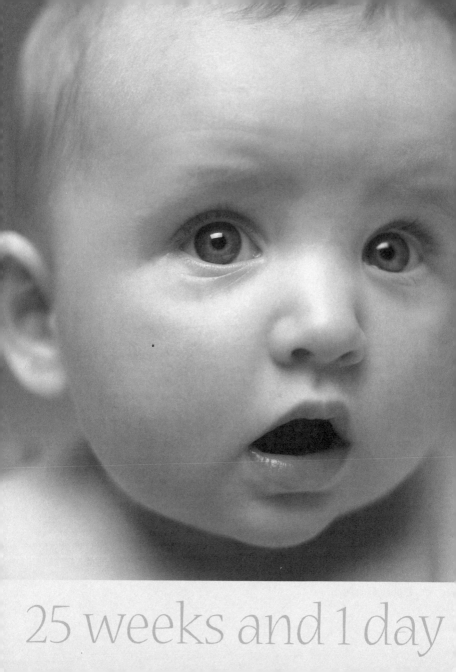

25 weeks and 1 day

104 days to go...

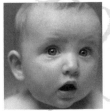

Did You Know?

A beautiful welcome present for your baby—and for you—could be to create a family tree. Expecting a child will certainly focus your mind on your own childhood and family life, and creating a family tree could be a satisfying way to explore these feelings. Talking to your immediate family is the best way to get started; then there are many excellent genealogy Web sites on the Internet.

WARNING

BECAUSE THEY ARE TINY, A BABY'S CORE TEMPERATURE WILL RISE FIVE TIMES MORE QUICKLY THAN THAT OF AN ADULT. ON A HOT DAY THE TEMPERATURE INSIDE A CAR WITHOUT AIR CONDITIONING CAN RISE, QUICKLY, CREATING A SERIOUS HEALTH RISK FOR A BABY.

Thoughts and Feelings...

....

....

....

....

....

....

....

....

....

DIARY DATES: ....

....

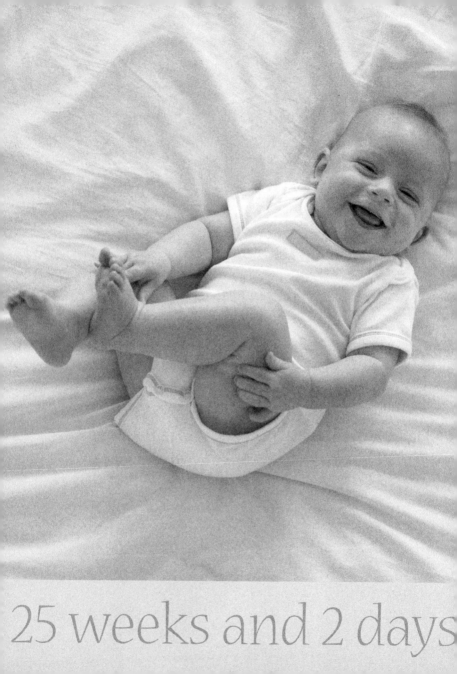

25 weeks and 2 days

103 days to go...

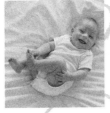

Giving Birth

It is unclear why some women become nauseous during dilation, especially in the transition phase as you reach full dilation. It is very difficult to absorb a contraction well, remain relaxed and vomit at the same time. If you are suffering from nausea, comfort yourself that it is probably related to the final stages of dilation, and that very soon you will be able to start pushing. Sometimes a change of position can help.

Thoughts and Feelings...

....

....

....

....

....

....

....

....

....

....

fact

Certain pain relief drugs will help you relax during labor, but they may also make your baby sleepy during birth and afterwards as well. Ask your care provider about any possible side effects.

DIARY DATES: ....

....

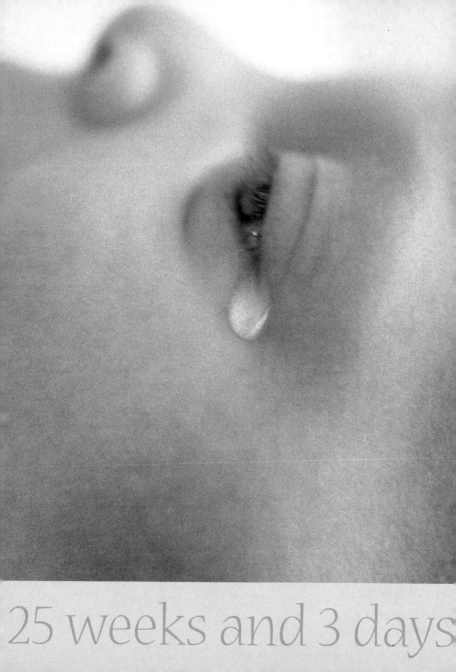

25 weeks and 3 days

102 days to go...

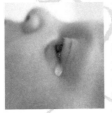

Health and Fitness

Leg and foot cramps may continue to be a problem and even become more severe as your pregnancy progresses and the blood circulation becomes slower than usual. They can be especially painful at night. A hot-water bottle against the calves can help, as can a pillow under the foot end of the mattress. Also try this gentle exercise that you can do whenever you are sitting down: stretch your leg and stretch your toes towards you.

Thoughts and Feelings...

....
....
....
....
....
....
....
....

WARNING

SCIATICA CAN CAUSE LEG CRAMPS. IT CAN ALSO CAUSE PAIN FROM YOUR BUTTOCKS DOWN THE LENGTH OF YOUR LEG. IF THE PAIN IS PERSISTENT TALK TO YOUR DOCTOR; A PHYSIOTHERAPIST MAY BE ABLE TO HELP RELIEVE THE PAIN.

DIARY DATES: ....
....

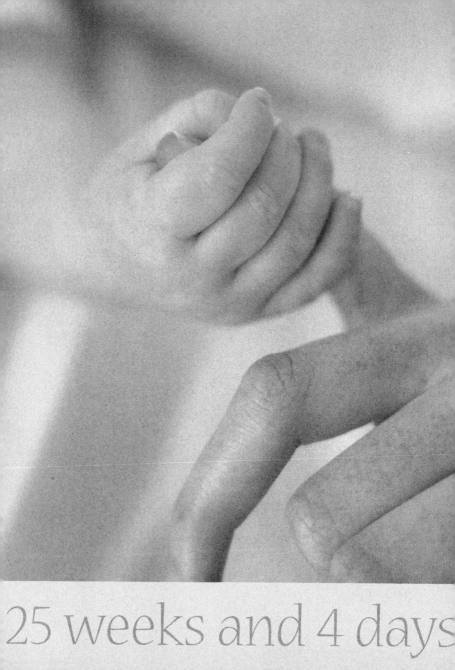

25 weeks and 4 days

101 days to go...

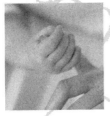

Baby's Development

The lungs reach an important stage of their development as more air sacs are produced, but they are only completely ready to function at the end of the eighth month. The transparent skin of the fetus is starting to thicken now, and sweat glands are being created below the surface of the skin. The baby is about 13in (33cm) in length and may weight around 2lb (0.9kg).

Thoughts and Feelings...

....

....

....

....

....

....

....

....

....

tip · tip

ONE OF THE ADVANTAGES OF BOTTLE FEEDING IS THAT SOMEONE ELSE CAN FEED YOUR BABY AS WELL AS YOU. IF YOU ARE BREASTFEEDING, YOU MAY WISH TO EXPRESS MILK SO YOUR PARTNER CAN GIVE THE LAST FEED OF THE DAY, ALLOWING YOU TO GET TO BED—READY FOR THE NIGHT FEEDS!

DIARY DATES: ....

....

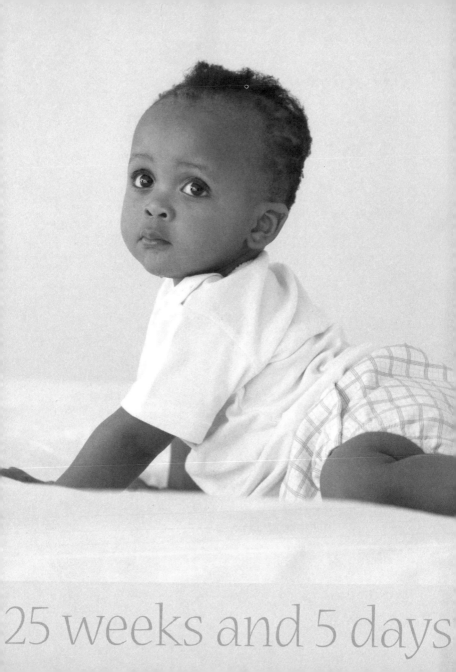
25 weeks and 5 days

100 days to go...

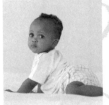

Did You Know?

There are a variety of parenting classes available. Most will tend to concentrate on the facts of labor and strategies for dealing with it. Classes are also a good opportunity for you to meet other expectant mothers in your area and share mutual anxieties. Your partner will be welcome at most of these classes. There are also classes that teach specific childbirth methods, such as Lamaze, which focus on breathing techniques.

"Mother knows what's best' always arouses bitterness in children."

Dame Agatha Christie, author (1890–1976)

fact

Frequently, free classes related to childbirth are available from your local hospital or various community organizations. Be sure to ask your care provider and other recent or expecting mothers if they are familiar with any such programs.

Thoughts and Feelings...

....
....
....
....
....
....

DIARY DATES: ....
....

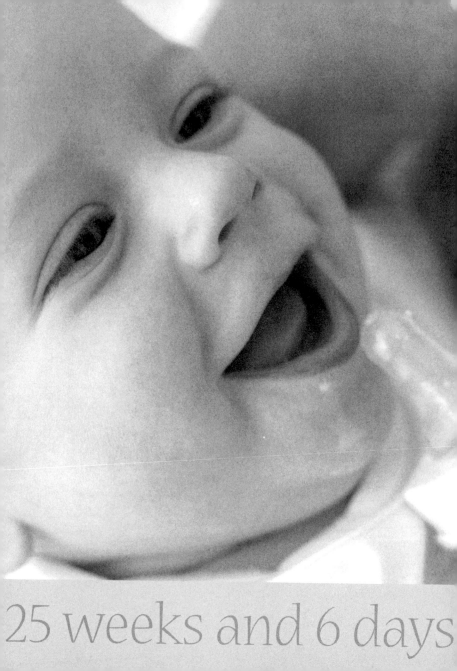

25 weeks and 6 days

99 days to go...

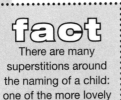

Baby Names for Boys

Malcolm (English)
Manfred (English)
Marcus (Latin)
Mark (English)
Marshall (French)
Martin (Latin)

Marvin (English)
Matthew (Hebrew)
Maurice (Latin)
Maxwell (Scottish)
Michael (Hebrew)
Murray (Scottish)

fact

There are many superstitions around the naming of a child: one of the more lovely trends that crosses many cultures is to name your child after nature, so that like a flower he or she will blossom and grow.

Thoughts and Feelings...

DIARY DATES: ....

....

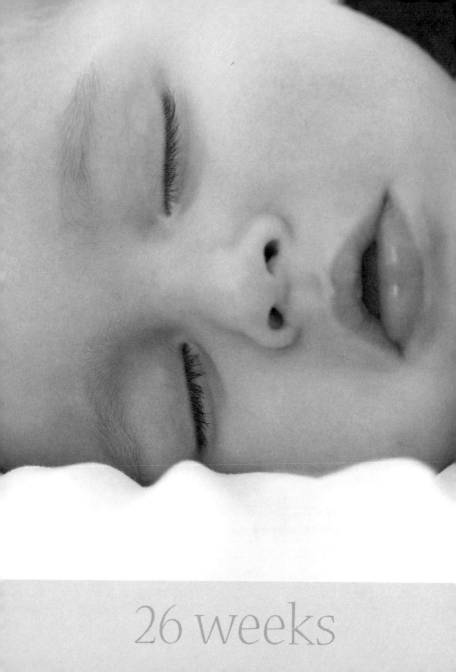

26 weeks

98 days to go...

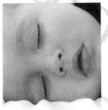

Your Pregnancy

Many women have trouble with varicose veins during their pregnancy. Valves in the legs are damaged by increased blood and pressure and the result is pooled blood in the veins of the lower leg. Varicose veins appear as fine red or blue lines and can cause considerable soreness in the legs. Wearing support stockings can help to relieve discomfort.

Thoughts and Feelings...

....

....

....

....

....

....

....

....

....

tip · tip

TRY TO KEEP CIRCULATION GOING BY CHANGING THE POSITION OF YOUR LEGS FREQUENTLY. REST ON THE LEFT SIDE AND TRY RAISING THE FOOT END OF YOUR BED SLIGHTLY. WHEN SITTING DOWN TRY TO KEEP YOUR FEET UP.

DIARY DATES: ....

....

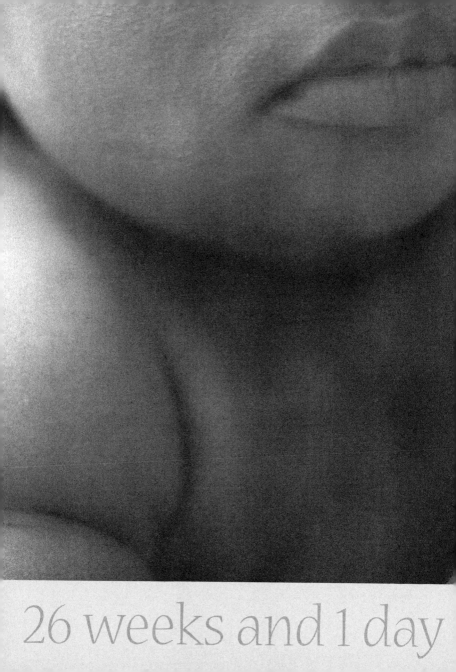

26 weeks and 1 day

97 days to go...

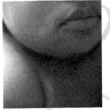

Did You Know?

More babies are born at full moon! Well, it may help to believe this if you are past your due date and the moon is looking very round, but unfortunately it is another old wives' tale. It probably grows out of the fact that it is hard to tell when the moon is truly full: if there is only a small slice missing the moon still looks pretty round.

Thoughts and Feelings...

....

....

....

....

....

....

....

....

....

....

....

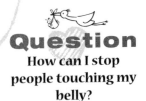

Question

How can I stop people touching my belly?

If people ask permission, you don't have to say yes. Tell them you are feeling sensitive about your stomach at the moment. If they don't ask, you can only rely on your powers of observation and manage to body-check them before they get to your stomach!

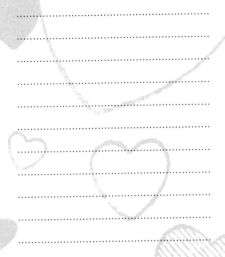

DIARY DATES: ....

....

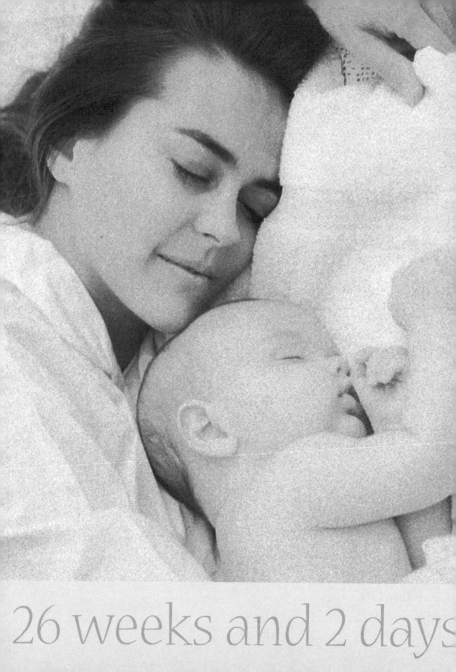

26 weeks and 2 days

96 days to go...

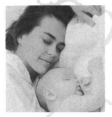

Giving Birth

The urge to push is caused by a reflexive impulse. An undulating urge comes from your stomach, making it virtually impossible for you not to push. The stomach muscles contract, together with a few other muscle groups, including the breathing muscles. The moment you are given the word to push from your doctor or midwife will probably come as a huge relief. The most effective moment to push is at the peak of a contraction.

Thoughts and Feelings...

....
....
....
....
....
....
....
....
....

reminder

If you find that grunting, moaning, or even screaming is an almost involuntary accompaniment to pushing, don't worry about it. Whatever it takes to work with your carer to get your baby delivered, is best at this point.

DIARY DATES: ....
....

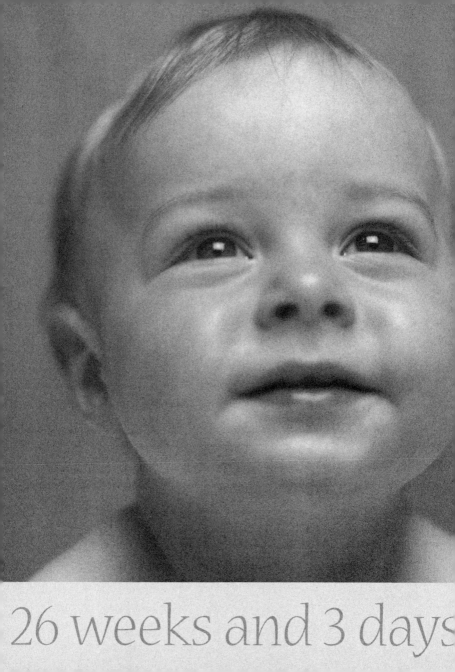

26 weeks and 3 days

95 days to go...

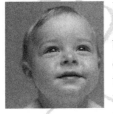

Health and Fitness

During pregnancy your nails may become brittle, and break or crack more easily. The cause of this is probably lack of iron. Reduce the use of nail polish because the polish only makes the nails weaker. It is better to use a nail-hardening cream. Boost iron intake by eating red meat or tofu, green leafy vegetables, dried apricots, seeds, and beans.

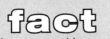

Your care provider may recommend an iron supplement, which comes in tablet, capsule, or oral liquid form. Iron supplements can cause nausea and other unpleasant side effects, so experiment with different forms as one may agree more with you than the other.

Thoughts and Feelings...

....
....
....
....
....
....
....
....
....
....

DIARY DATES: ....
....

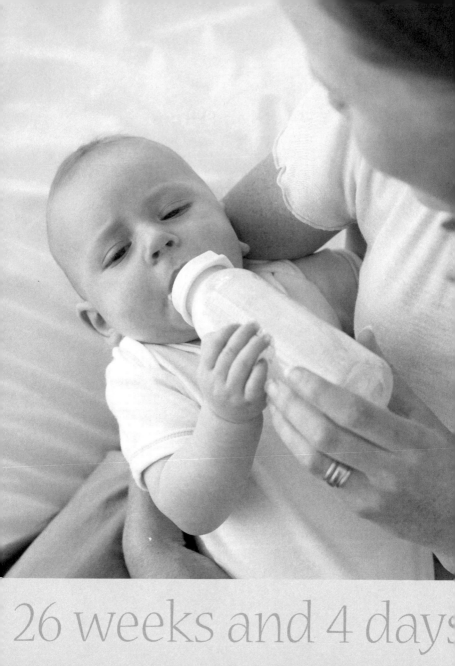

26 weeks and 4 days

94 days to go...

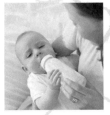

Baby's Development

More and more fat is stored in the baby's body now, and this fat will help to regulate her body temperature now and after birth. Her small heart is beating about twice as fast as the mother's heart. In the case of a boy, the number of testosterone-producing cells in the testicles is starting to increase. The baby is roughly 13⅜in (34cm) in length, and there is less room for her to manoeuvre insider your womb now.

Thoughts and Feelings...

....
....
....
....
....
....
....
....
....

reminder

If this is your second baby and you had problems breastfeeding the first time around, don't be put off from trying again. New experiences can be particularly stressful and this time you will have experience on your side: plus a different baby.

DIARY DATES: ....

....

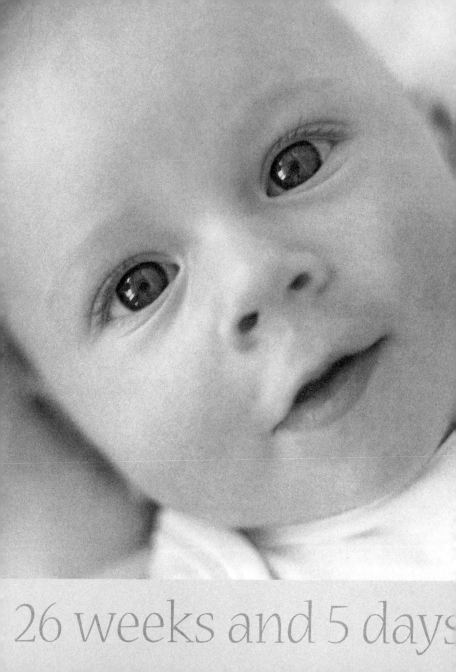

26 weeks and 5 days

93 days to go...

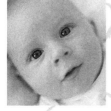

Did You Know?

An epidural is an effective form of pain relief: it is injected into the space between your spinal column and the spinal cord by an anasthesiologist. It is possible to have a mobile dose, which allows you to move around. Your dose will probably need to be increased as labor progresses. An epidural may also be used for Cesarean section, allowing the mother to be awake during

Thoughts and Feelings...

....
....
....
....
....
....
....
....
....
....

fact

A TENS machine sends a weak electrical current to the brain, blocking pain sensations and encouraging the release of the pain-suppressing hormone endorphins. You may be able to rent a machine in advance of labor.

DIARY DATES: ....
....

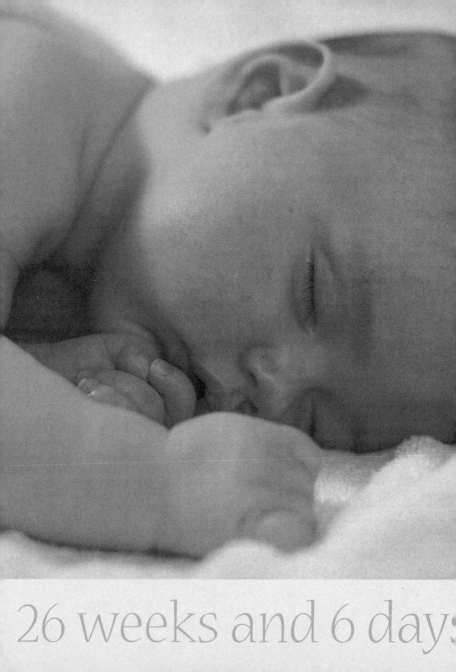

26 weeks and 6 day:

92 days to go...

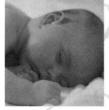

Baby Names for Girls

Nadia (Russian)   Nicole (English)
Nancy (Hebrew)   Nina (Spanish)
Naomi (Hebrew)   Noel (French)
Natalie (Latin)   Nora (Greek)
Natasha (Russian)   Norma (Latin)

fact

	was born as...	
Billy Idol		William Broad
Cary Grant		Archibald Leach
Bruce Lee		Lee Yuen Kam
Sophia Loren		Sofia Scicolone
Freddy Mercury		Farokh Bulsara

Thoughts and Feelings...

....
....
....
....
....

DIARY DATES: ....
....

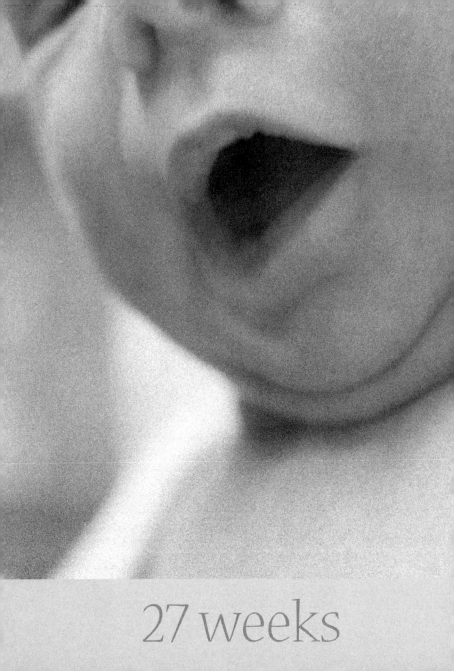

27 weeks

91 days to go...

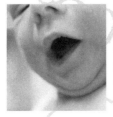

Your Pregnancy

During this stage it is good to start thinking about the many pieces of equipment you may want to purchase for the baby. These will range from changing mats, baby bath, and nail scissors to major items such as a stroller, a car seat, and somewhere for the baby to sleep. You will probably need at least three changes of clothes per day when they are tiny, so remember to check the washing instructions of any clothes you buy.

Thoughts and Feelings...

....
....
....
....
....
....
....
....
....
....

reminder

Be sure to ask friends who have children if they have any equipment they can pass on or sell to you. It is also worth checking charity shops and small ads in the local newspaper for all sorts of baby equipment if you want to keep costs down.

Diary Dates: ....

....

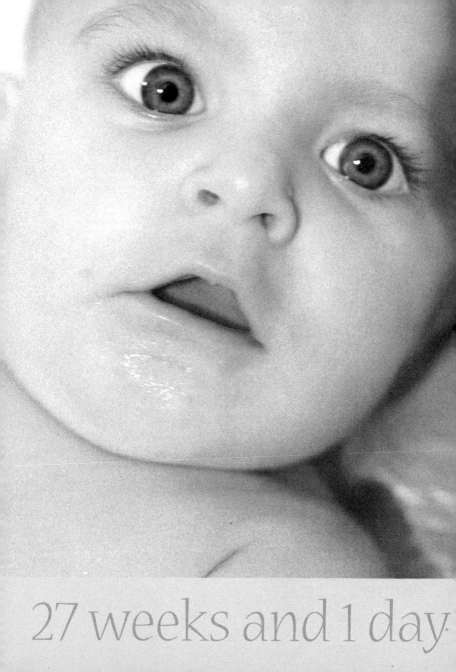

27 weeks and 1 day

90 days to go...

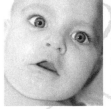

Did You Know?

You may be able to take advantage of a birthing tub at your hospital or birthing center. This will enable you to spend part of your labor in warm water, which can help you to relax and ease the discomfort of contractions. Some women choose to deliver the baby into water, but you must ensure your care provider is aware you wish to do this, and also that it is allowed by the regulations of your hospital or birthing center.

Thoughts and Feelings...

....

....

....

....

....

....

....

....

....

tip · tip

MUSIC MAY ENCOURAGE OR DISTRACT YOU DURING LABOUR. HOWEVER, IT IS LIKELY THAT OTHER WOMEN WILL BE IN LABOUR NEARBY SO YOU WILL EITHER HAVE TO KEEP THE VOLUME DOWN OR USE EARPHONES (WHICH WILL MEAN BEING ATTACHED TO YET ANOTHER PIECE OF ELECTRICAL EQUIPMENT).

DIARY DATES: ....

....

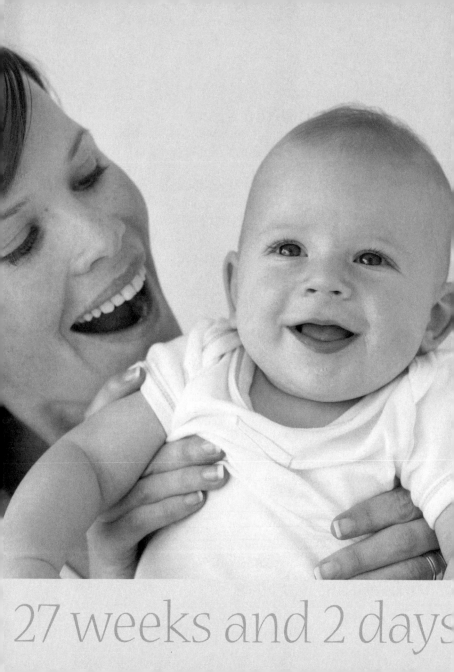

27 weeks and 2 days

89 days to go...

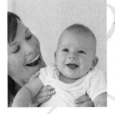

Giving Birth

The bottom of the pelvis is strong and does not give much when you are trying to push the baby out. The baby's head will then have to turn a bit to make the birth possible, and it is at this point that a tear may occur at the opening of the vagina. If your care provider thinks a tear is inevitable they will suggest an episiotomy, making a small cut, instead.

Thoughts and Feelings...

....

....

....

....

....

....

....

....

....

....

fact

After the delivery of the placenta, any stitches you need to repair a tear or episiotomy will be given. If you have not used pain relief, a local anaesthetic may be administered to numb the area.

DIARY DATES: ....

....

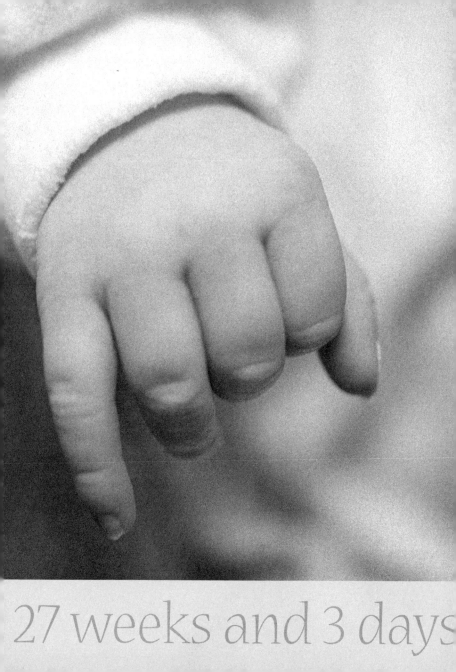

27 weeks and 3 days

88 days to go...

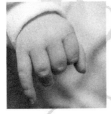

Health and Fitness

Discuss any holiday plans with your care provider or doctor. Airline companies apply certain restrictions concerning how far into the pregnancy a woman is still allowed to fly with them: some do not wish to carry women over 28 weeks pregnant because of the risk of premature labor. Others will require a medical certificate stating you are fit to travel. In general, it is advisable not to fly from the seventh month on.

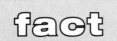

As your pregnancy progresses you may suffer from mild shortness of breath, headaches, forgetfulness, water retention, breast tenderness, cramp, backache, frequent urination, bleeding gums, excess mucus and saliva, increase in vaginal discharge, gas and heartburn—as well as fatigue.

Thoughts and Feelings...

....

....

....

....

....

....

....

....

....

....

DIARY DATES: ....

....

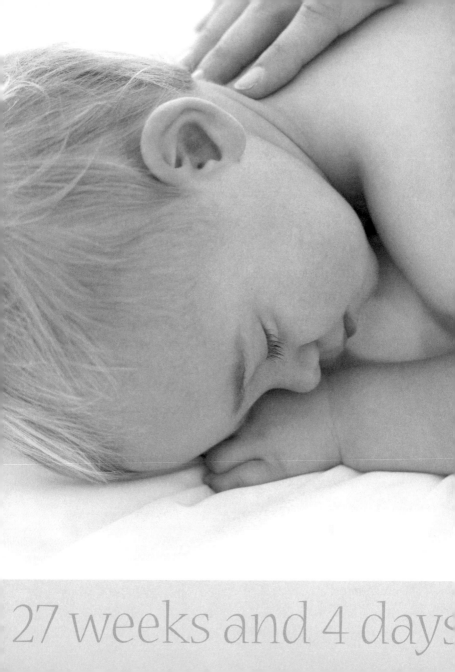

27 weeks and 4 days

87 days to go...

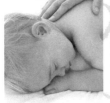

Baby's Development

The baby is growing amazingly fast at this stage. Although he may be moving slightly less, you will be conscious of the movements and as well as feeling them you may begin to see them too. It is a remarkable experience to see your baby's limbs punching out of your skin. He is practising sucking now and may even be seen sucking a thumb or fist on an ultrasound scan. Baby is roughly 13¾in (35cm) long now.

Thoughts and Feelings...

....
....
....
....
....
....
....
....
....
....

fact

The lungs are developing, but would still be unable to function in the outside world. If an early delivery were called for, steroids might be given intravenously to boost lung development at the last minute.

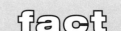

DIARY DATES: ....
....

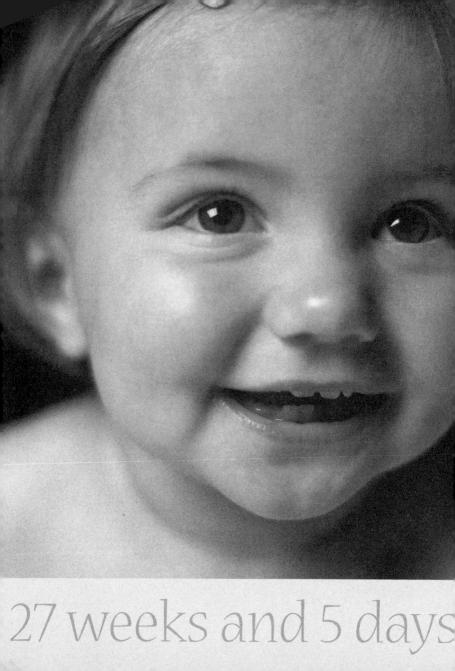

27 weeks and 5 days

86 days to go...

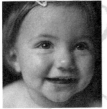

Did You Know?

In recent decades, the average age of mothers has increased, as women marry later on average, delay becoming pregnant for career or other reasons, and have children more frequently in their 40s (partly due to advances in reproductive technology). There are pros and cons to being a younger or older mother. Younger women may have more energy but less money, while older women report feeling more ready for motherhood emotionally.

"Of course it's difficult, but the younger mothers in my help group have it tough as well."

Diane Keaton, actress, speaking about late motherhood

(she adopted her daughter, Dexter, at the age of 49 (taken from *Beau Monde*))

Thoughts and Feelings...

....

....

....

....

....

....

fact

Older mothers may be more financially secure, but as well as caring for small children they may have to carry the burden of caring for their own older parents.

DIARY DATES: ....

....

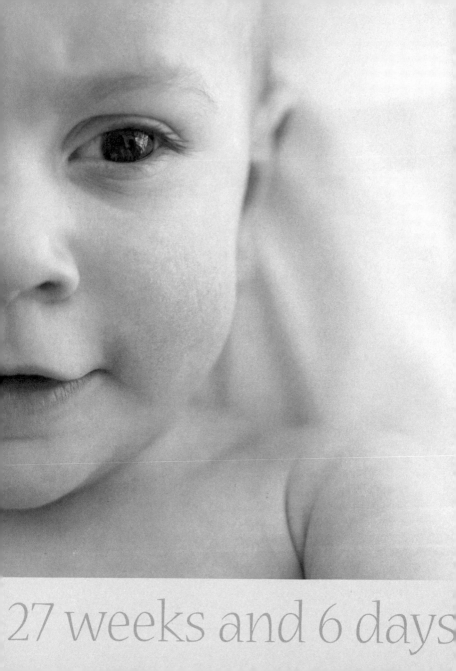

27 weeks and 6 days

85 days to go...

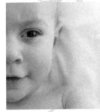

Baby Names for Boys

Nathan (Hebrew)
Neil (Irish)
Nevin (Irish)
Nicholas (Greek)
Nigel (Irish)

Noah (Hebrew)
Nolan (Irish)
Norman (English)
Norton (English)
Nye (Welsh)

Thoughts and Feelings...

....
....
....
....
....
....
....
....
....
....
....

tip · tip

AS MORE AND MORE PEOPLE CHOOSE TO KNOW THE SEX OF THEIR BABY BEFORE DELIVERY DAY, IT IS POSSIBLE TO FIX ON A NAME EARLY ON IN THE PREGNANCY. THIS CAN HELP YOU TO BOND WITH THE BABY, IF YOU START TO TALK TO HIM OR HER BY NAME.

DIARY DATES: ....

....

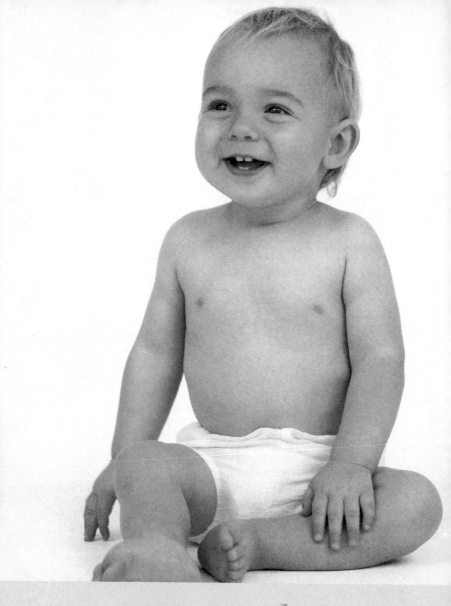

28 weeks

84 days to go...

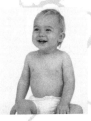

Your Pregnancy

You are developing quite a belly now: the fundus is halfway between your belly button and your breastbone and it is pushing on your stomach, intestines and diaphragm. In this last trimester, many expectant women have one dream after another about babies and giving birth, and some of these dreams can be unpleasant. Your conscious and unconscious fears and doubts are rising to the surface, and this is one way of dealing with them.

Thoughts and Feelings...

....
....
....
....
....
....
....
....
....

reminder

Sharing anxieties can reduce them: talk to your partner about your fears and if you know other women who are pregnant plan a get-together so you can all let off steam together.

DIARY DATES: .....Routine check-up...

....

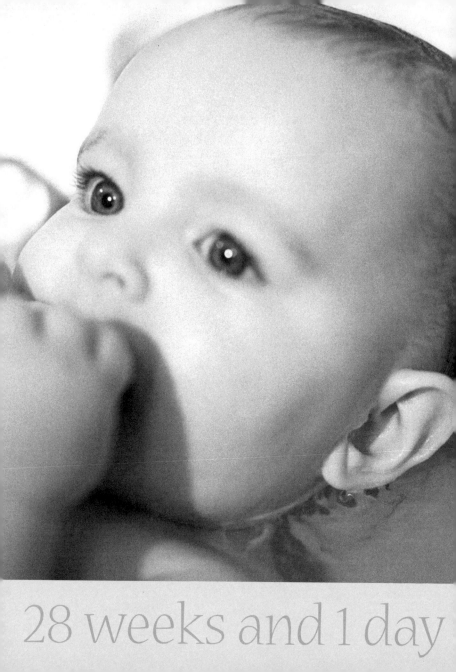

28 weeks and 1 day

83 days to go...

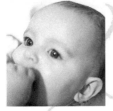

Did You Know?

Women who wear contact lenses or glasses may have problems during their pregnancy. Fluid retention causes the eyeball to retain more moisture, which can lead to the cornea changing shape and create minor changes in vision. Estrogen, on the other hand, causes the eye to dry out and if you wear contact lenses this can lead to soreness and irritation.

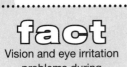

fact

Vision and eye irritation problems during pregnancy are most likely temporary. Investing in new corrective lenses could be expensive; try to manage until after the birth and you will probably find the problem corrects itself.

Thoughts and Feelings...

....
....
....
....
....
....
....
....
....

DIARY DATES: ....

....

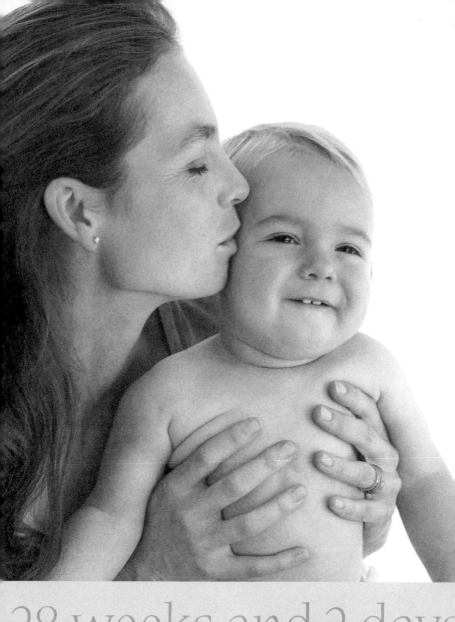

28 weeks and 2 days

82 days to go...

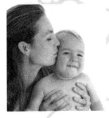

Giving Birth

The chances of tearing, or needing an episiotomy, can be substantially reduced by following the instructions of your doctor, nurse, or midwife. She will advise you—at the moment the head appears—to absorb the contractions with the aid of your breathing and not to push along with your stomach muscles. She may also try perineal massage with Vitamin E oil or another lubricant or warm compresses to avoid

Thoughts and Feelings...

....

....

....

....

....

....

....

....

tip · tip ·

IF YOU ARE DETERMINED NOT TO HAVE AN EPISIOTOMY, YOU NEED TO INCLUDE THIS IN YOUR BIRTH PLAN SO YOUR DOCTOR AND MIDWIFE ARE AWARE OF YOUR WISHES. HOWEVER, YOU ALSO NEED TO ACCEPT THAT EMERGENCIES HAPPEN, AND IF THE BABY IS IN DISTRESS MEDICAL STAFF WILL ACT TO GET THE BABY OUT QUICKLY.

DIARY DATES: ....

....

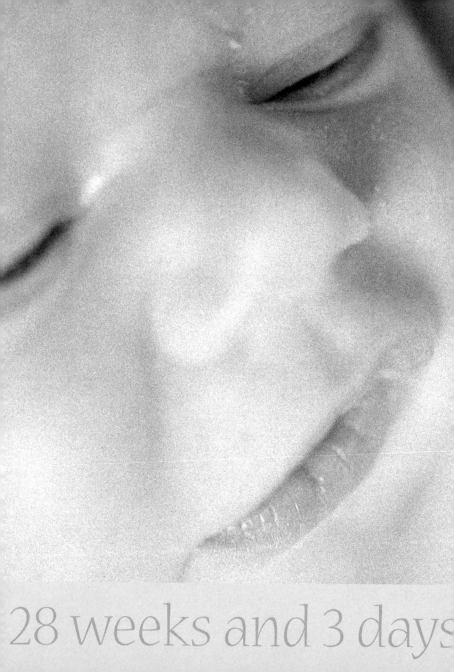

28 weeks and 3 days

81 days to go...

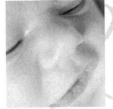

Health and Fitness

You are likely to need a larger size bra towards the end of your pregnancy. You may choose a supportive nursing bra if you plan to breastfeed. Choose a bra with a broad band under the cups and wide, adjustable straps. If you are due to deliver in the summer, buy a cotton or cotton-blend bra that will breathe and be more comfortable in hot weather. You may also find it more comfortable to wear your bra in bed during the last few months.

Thoughts and Feelings...

....
....
....
....
....
....
....
....

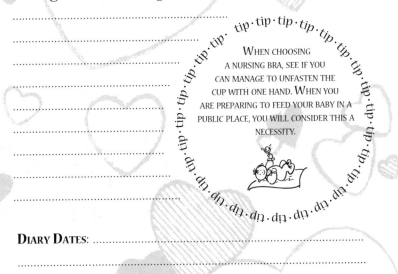

tip · tip

WHEN CHOOSING A NURSING BRA, SEE IF YOU CAN MANAGE TO UNFASTEN THE CUP WITH ONE HAND. WHEN YOU ARE PREPARING TO FEED YOUR BABY IN A PUBLIC PLACE, YOU WILL CONSIDER THIS A NECESSITY.

DIARY DATES: ....
....

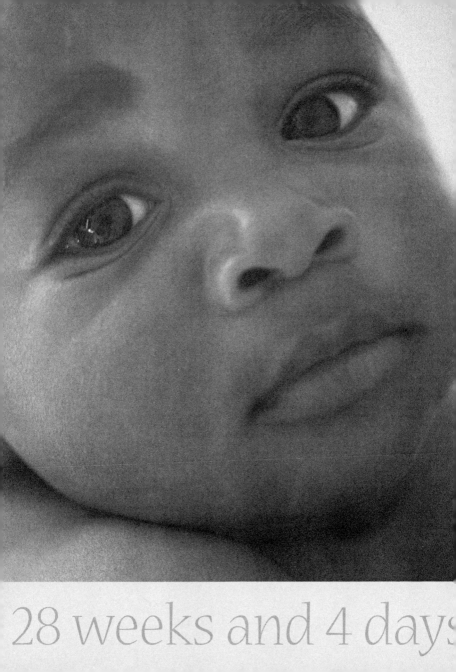

28 weeks and 4 days

80 days to go...

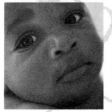

Baby's Development

The baby's eyes are fully open now, and she has a dim view of her surroundings, and is able to sense light filtering through the skin of your abdomen. Her breathing exercises are more and more controlled. Her stomach and intestines are functioning; the kidneys are almost formed, but will not be completely in order until after the birth. She is now 14⅜in (36.5cm) long.

Thoughts and Feelings...

....

....

....

....

....

....

....

....

....

....

THE DIGESTIVE SYSTEM OF A NEWBORN BABY CAN ONLY COPE WITH 2–4TSP (10–20ML) OF BREAST OR BOTTLE MILK AND YOU MAY NOTICE SPITTING UP—THIS IS USUALLY JUST OVERSPILL. IF IT IS EXCESSIVE OR PROJECTILE, CONTACT YOUR DOCTOR.

DIARY DATES: ....

....

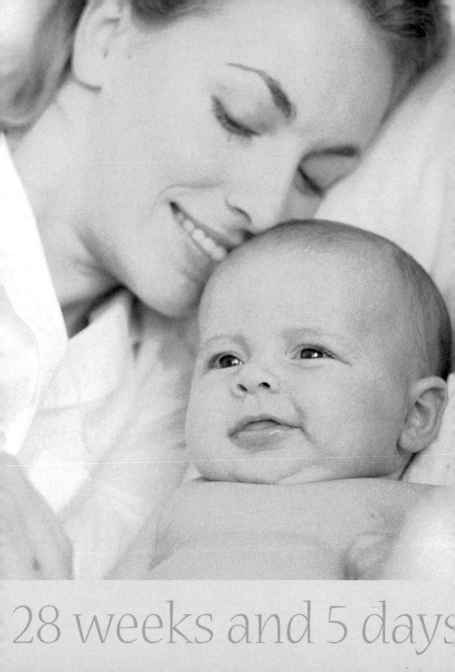

28 weeks and 5 days

79 days to go...

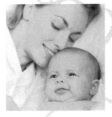

Did You Know?

Newborn babies enjoy frequent feeding. Fussy feeding can sometimes indicate hunger; however, if the baby produces six to eight wet diapers and three dirty diapers daily then things are fine. If you are breastfeeding, these frequent snacks can help to stimulate your milk supply, which will then be sufficient as the baby grows and wants to eat larger amounts at once, but less frequently.

Thoughts and Feelings...

....

....

....

....

....

....

....

....

....

....

fact

If you have multiples you may want to establish a feeding routine sooner rather than later. You could try waiting until one baby wakes to feed, then waking the other baby or babies to feed at the same time; this will maximize your rest time between feeds.

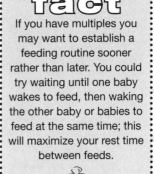

DIARY DATES: ....

....

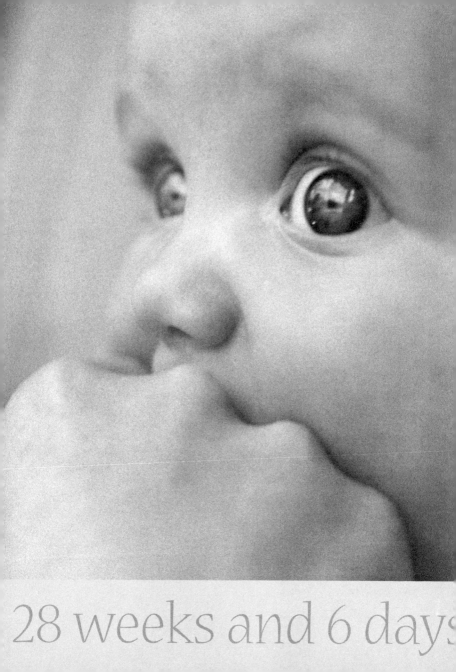

28 weeks and 6 days

78 days to go…

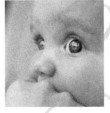

Baby Names for Girls

Octavia (Latin)
Odette (French)
Olga (Russian)
Olivia (Latin)
Oona (Irish)
Opal (English)

Ophelia (Greek)
Oprah (African American)
Oralie (French)
Oriana (Latin)

Thoughts and Feelings…

....
....
....
....
....
....
....
....
....
....

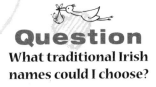

Question

What traditional Irish names could I choose?

BOYS	GIRLS
· Aichill	· Aifric
· Brendan	· Maire
· Clarán	· Ranait
· Kenneth	· Róis
· Seán	· Sinéad

DIARY DATES: ....
....

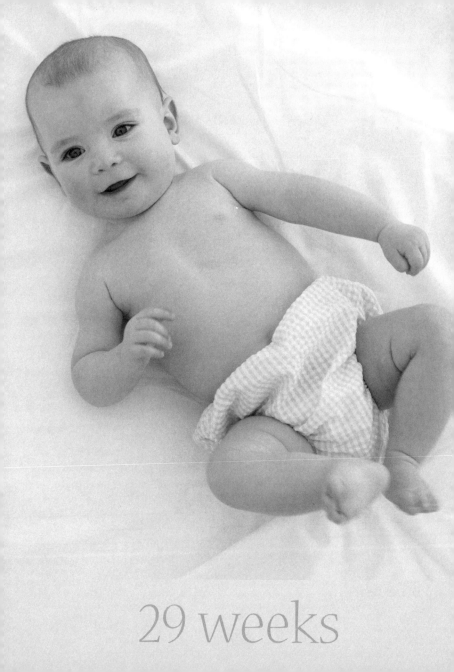

29 weeks

77 days to go...

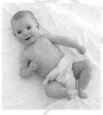

Your Pregnancy

Your womb is putting quite a bit of pressure on your bladder, as a result of which the bladder can hold less urine than usual. In addition, your body is retaining more salt and water, and the result is constant visits to the bathroom—both day and night. You may even find yourself dribbling urine when you sneeze or laugh, the result of stress incontinence. Make sure you do your pelvic floor exercises.

WARNING

A STEADY FLOW OF LIQUID MAY BE AMNIOTIC FLUID. THIS WILL BE CLEAR TO STRAW COLORED (OR POSSIBLY TINGED GREEN OR BROWN) AND HAVE A FAINTLY SWEET SMELL. TELL YOUR DOCTOR IMMEDIATELY, AS IT COULD INDICATE THAT YOUR MEMBRANES HAVE RUPTURED AND LEAD TO INFECTION.

Thoughts and Feelings...

....
....
....
....
....
....
....
....

DIARY DATES: ....

....

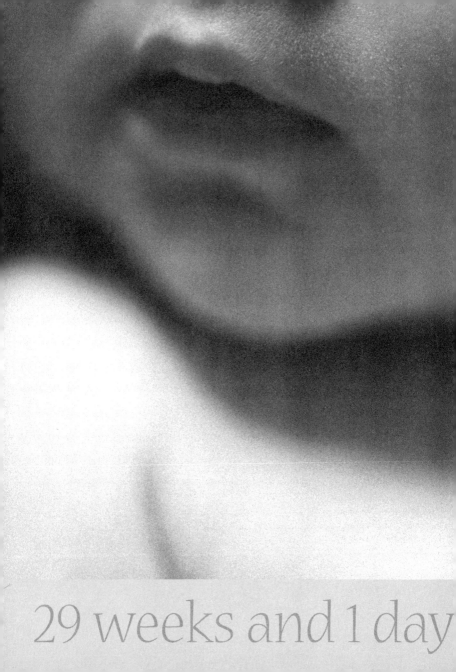

29 weeks and 1 day

76 days to go…

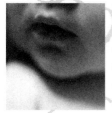

Did You Know?

Taking your baby into bed with you can be comforting for baby and a beautiful bonding experience for both parents. However, there are risks. In the United States, about 64 children die each year due to suffocation or crushing in the parental bed. A baby can be trapped between the mattress and the wall or be crushed by parents due to exhaustion, or the consumption of alcohol or tranquillizers.

Thoughts and Feelings…

....
....
....
....
....
....
....
....
....

WARNING

IF YOU HAVE A WATERBED, NEVER BRING YOUR BABY TO SLEEP WITH YOU IN IT. IF THEY LIE ON THEIR STOMACHS THEY WILL SINK INTO THE BED AND BE DEPRIVED OF AIR, LEADING TO SUFFOCATION. NEVER SLEEP ON A SOFA WITH A BABY, AS AGAIN THEY RISK SUFFOCATION OR FALLING FROM THE EDGE OF THE SOFA.

DIARY DATES: ....

....

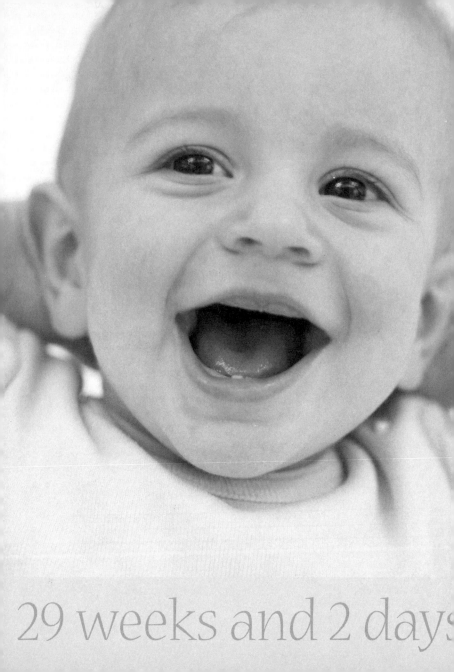

29 weeks and 2 days

75 days to go...

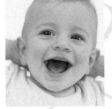

Giving Birth

A major anxiety as the day of childbirth approaches may be how you will cope with the pain. Many women find they are able to endure the pain; many other women decide, either before the day or as the pain of childbirth is actually experienced, that they need some assistance in the form of pain relief. Attending childbirth classes and understanding the nature of the pain will help you deal with it better on the day.

Thoughts and Feelings...

....

....

....

....

....

....

....

....

....

tip · tip

MANY WOMEN ARE FINDING ALTERNATIVE PAIN RELIEF METHODS SUCH AS ACUPUNCTURE, REFLEXOLOGY, AROMATHERAPY MASSAGE AND HYPNOSIS HELPFUL. YOU WILL NEED A PROFESSIONAL PRACTITIONER TO HELP YOU, AS WELL AS THE PERMISSION OF YOUR HOSPITAL OR BIRTH CENTER.

DIARY DATES: ....

....

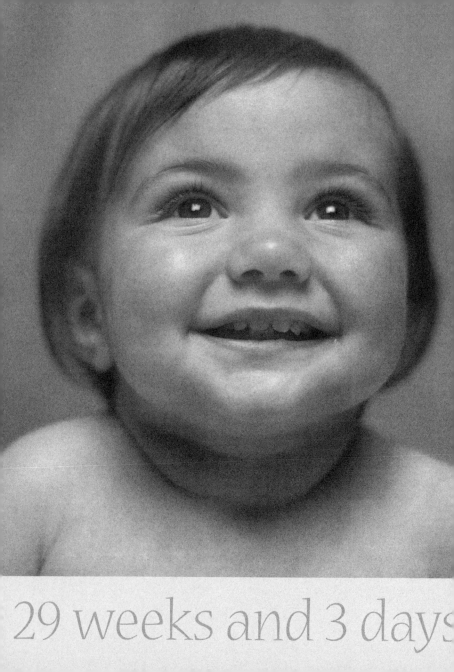

29 weeks and 3 days

74 days to go...

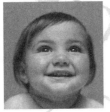

Health and Fitness

Shoes should be comfortable, but they shouldn't be too big, as they need to offer sturdy support. The best thing is a small heel or a solid, raised sole and possibly the use of support hose. If you work on your feet for long periods of time, try to move and change position as often as possible. To help relieve foot aches, alternate a hot and cold footbath, followed by a massage with foot cream or oil.

Thoughts and Feelings...

....
....
....
....
....
....
....
....
....

WARNING

A SEATED JOB CAN HAVE ITS OWN DISCOMFORTS. GET UP AND MOVE AROUND AS OFTEN AS POSSIBLE. USE A CUSHION TO SUPPORT YOUR BACK AND TRY TO RAISE YOUR FEET UNDER THE DESK — USE A PILE OF BOOKS IF NOTHING ELSE IS AVAILABLE.

DIARY DATES: ....
....

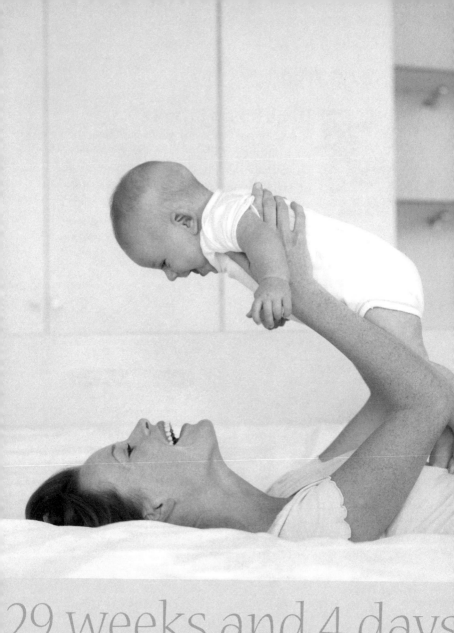

29 weeks and 4 days

73 days to go...

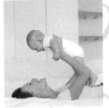

Baby's Development

The baby has grown so much that she is filling almost all of the space in the womb. Because of the lack of room you may feel her moving slightly less. The small skeleton is also changing, as the cartilage continues to ossify so that the bones will already be relatively firm at birth. Baby is roughly 15in (38cm) in length.

WARNING

TO REDUCE THE RISK OF SUDDEN INFANT DEATH SYNDROME ALWAYS PLACE SMALL BABIES TO SLEEP ON THEIR BACK. THEIR FEET SHOULD TOUCH THE BOTTOM OF THE COT OR BASKET AND COVERINGS SHOULD BE TUCKED IN AND COME NO HIGHER THAN THE BABY'S CHEST. REMOVE SOFT TOYS.

Thoughts and Feelings...

....

....

....

....

....

....

....

....

DIARY DATES: ....

....

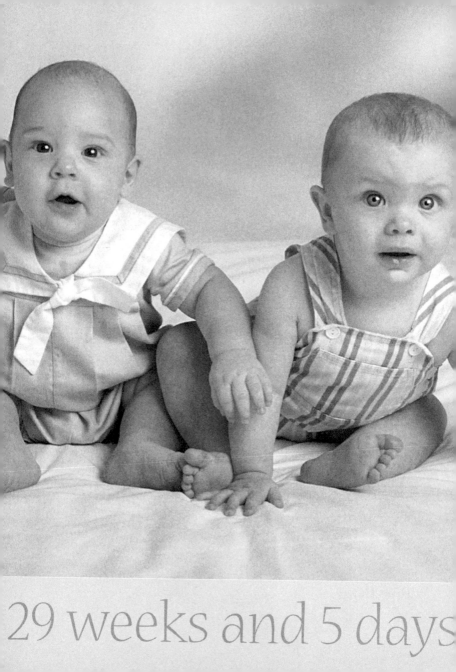

29 weeks and 5 days

72 days to go...

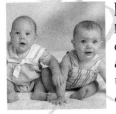

Did You Know?

Many factors will influence your decision on how much maternity leave to take and in what capacity you wish to return to work. Money will be very important, of course, along with your company's policy on maternity leave. The company's general attitude towards pregnancy and working mothers will also influence your thinking. If you don't want to return quickly, or in a full-time capacity, try to think of creative alternatives and approach your boss early in your pregnancy.

Thoughts and Feelings...

....

....

....

....

....

....

....

....

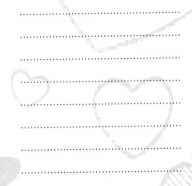

"If I ever got the chance to have children, I'd want to devote all of my time and attention to them. I'd want to give them a happy and secure youth with a fantastic mom and dad...But I don't know if that's how it's going to be or what the future has in store for me."

Mariah Carey, singer (taken from *Viva*)

DIARY DATES: ....

....

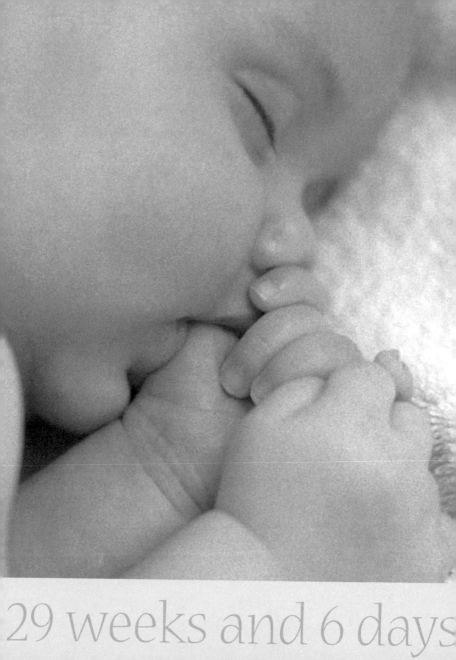

29 weeks and 6 days

71 days to go...

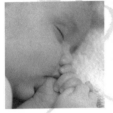

Baby Names for Girls

Page (French)
Pamela (Greek)
Paris (Greek)
Patience (English)
Patricia (English)
Paula (Latin)

Pearl (Latin)
Penelope (Greek)
Philippa (Greek)
Phoebe (Greek)
Polly (English)
Priscilla (English)

fact

George Michael   was born as...   Giorgios Panayiotou
Marilyn Monroe   Norma Jean Baker
Edith Piaf   Edith Gassion
Françoise Sagan   Françoise Quoirez
Romy Schneider   Rosemarie Albach-Retty

Thoughts and Feelings...

....

....

....

....

....

DIARY DATES: ....

....

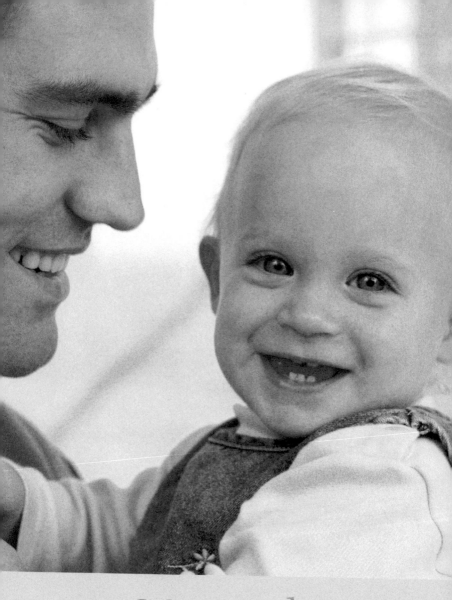

30 weeks

30 weeks

70 days to go...

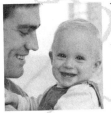

Your Pregnancy

Your baby may soon start to move into the vertex, or head-down, position. However, if you feel a lot of kicking on your pelvic floor it is likely that the baby is still sitting or standing upright. Alternatively, he could be lying across your womb in a transverse position. If a breech position is suspected, your doctor or care provider will probably use a scan closer to your due date to confirm the baby's position.

Thoughts and Feelings...

....

....

....

....

....

....

....

....

fact

Your care provider may try a manual technique called external cephalic version to turn your baby. This is successful in about 50% of instances. It shouldn't be attempted too far in advance of your due date, as the baby may simply turn back again.

DIARY DATES: ....

....

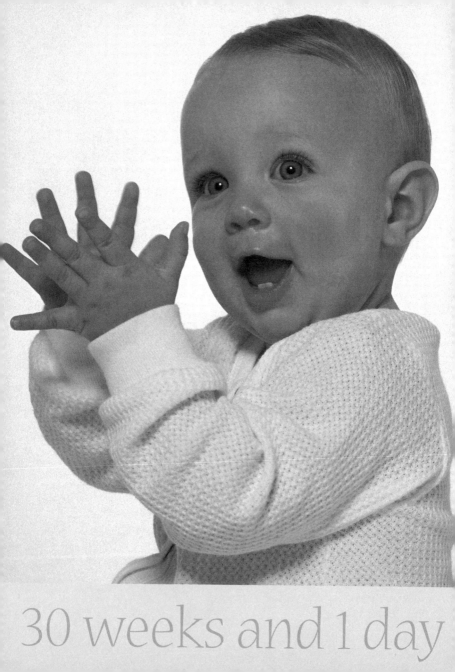

30 weeks and 1 day

69 days to go...

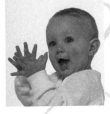

Did You Know?

Whether you have wide or narrow hips has nothing to do with the ease with which you give birth. A problem arises if a baby has a disproportionately large head or the mother fails to fully dilate. If baby needs help to exit the birth canal, forceps may be used. This tong-like device is used to grasp the baby's head and pull him free. They can also be used to reposition baby.

Thoughts and Feelings...

....
....
....
....
....
....
....
....

WARNING

THE USE OF FORCEPS TO AID IN DELIVERY CAN LEAVE MARKS ON A NEWBORN. THE BABY MAY BE BRUISED ON EITHER SIDE OF THE HEAD FOR A FEW DAYS. THERE IS ALSO A VERY SLIM RISK OF BRAIN INJURY.

DIARY DATES: ....

....

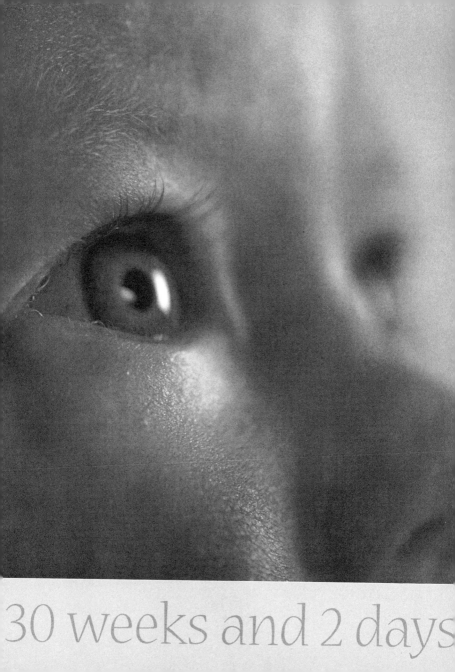

30 weeks and 2 days

68 days to go...

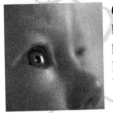

Giving Birth

Delivery by Cesarean section may be planned, or it may happen as an emergency procedure after a difficult labor. If it is planned, you will probably be offered an epidural, which will allow you to be awake when your baby is born. If it is unscheduled, you may well be given a general anesthetic that will render you unconscious. If you are conscious at the moment of birth, your baby will quickly be cleaned and checked over, then passed straight to you.

Thoughts and Feelings...

....
....
....
....
....
....
....
....

Question

How will a Cesarean effect me?

A Cesarean counts as major surgery and you will be advised to lift nothing heavier than your new baby for six weeks afterwards. Painkillers are given to alleviate any discomfort, and the stitches will not deter you from nursing and bonding with your baby.

DIARY DATES: ....
....

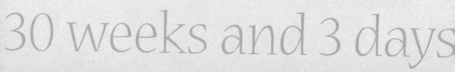
30 weeks and 3 days

67 days to go...

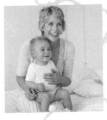

Health and Fitness

Finishing your shower by spraying hot then cold water on to your breasts is good for strengthening the breast tissue. Massage the nipples forcefully while drying yourself and then softly rub cream, oil or lotion on the skin. No matter what your breast or nipple size you will, in all likelihood, breastfeed successfully.

Thoughts and Feelings...

....

....

....

....

....

....

....

....

....

tip · tip ·

EVEN IF YOU HAVE HAD YOUR NIPPLES PIERCED YOU MAY BE ABLE TO BREASTFEED. HOWEVER, SOME PIERCINGS CAN SCAR THE MILK DUCTS, AND IF YOU HAVE HAD AN INFECTED PIERCING OR HAVE MULTIPLE PIERCINGS YOU MAY HAVE MORE DIFFICULTY.

DIARY DATES: ....

....

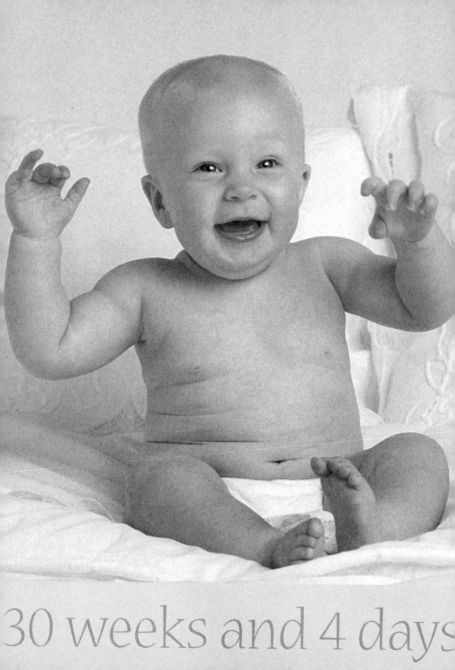

30 weeks and 4 days

66 days to go...

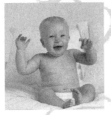

Baby's Development

Most of the organs are now fully developed, although the lungs still need time to come to maturity—outside the womb your baby would still be unable to breath unassisted. The baby can feel pain now and responds to pressure from the outside and also startles easily at loud noises. The baby is now roughly 15½in (39cm) in length.

Thoughts and Feelings...

....

....

....

....

....

....

....

....

....

....

fact

Your baby's eyelashes and eyebrows are fully grown now. His eyes open and close, and his eyesight is beginning to come into focus. He is developing a full head of hair, and this will continue to grow up to delivery day.

DIARY DATES: ....

....

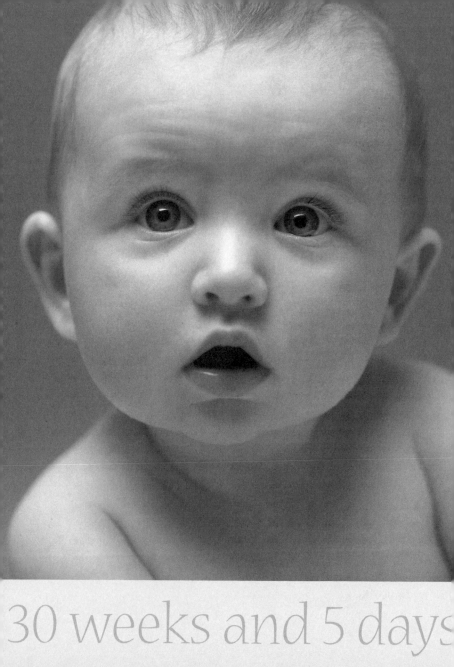

30 weeks and 5 days

65 days to go...

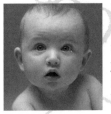

Did You Know?

If you have children already, give them time to adjust to the idea of a new sibling. When you break the news, instant excitement may not be the response you get. Try to keep life on an even keel, although some hurdles are unavoidable. If your older child has to face a challenge, such as starting at a new school, make sure the big event is given the attention it warrants.

Thoughts and Feelings...

....

....

....

....

....

....

....

....

....

"To be honest, I find non-pregnant bodies much more beautiful. I look in the mirror and pray that the best parts of me won't be gone after I've had a baby."

Cindy Crawford, top model (taken from *Beau Monde*)

DIARY DATES: ....

....

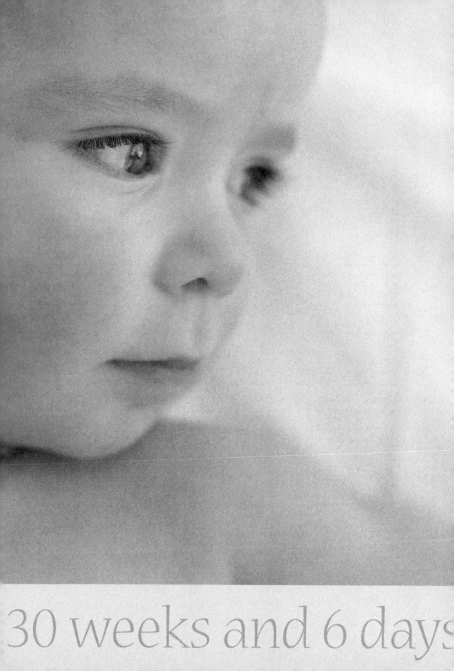
30 weeks and 6 days

64 days to go...

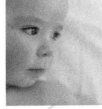

Baby Names for Boys

Patrick (Irish)   Phelan (Irish)
Paul (Latin)   Philip (Greek)
Percy (English)   Phineas (Hebrew)
Peter (Greek)   Prescott (English)

WARNING

TAKE CARE TO CONSIDER WHAT THE INITIALS OF YOUR CHOSEN NAME SPELL OUT. KIDS WILL PICK UP ON THE SLIGHTEST DETAIL, SO SAVE YOUR CHILD SOME HEARTACHE IN THE FUTURE AND GIVE THESE LETTERS A GOOD HARD LOOK!

Thoughts and Feelings...

....
....
....
....
....
....
....
....
....

DIARY DATES: ....

....

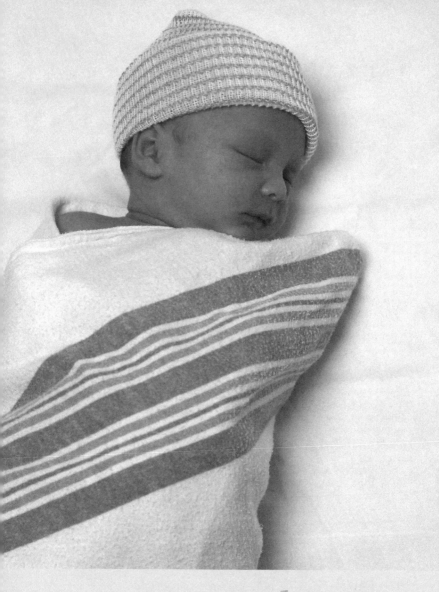

31 weeks

31 weeks

63 days to go...

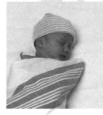

Your Pregnancy

As the available space is reduced, the number of baby movements will reduce. Make a note of your baby's pattern of activity—for instance, she may sleep in the mornings and be livelier in the afternoon and evening. If you don't feel any movements, or a dramatically reduced number of movements over the course of 24 hours, you should contact your doctor.

Thoughts and Feelings...

....

....

....

....

....

....

....

....

....

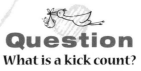

Question
What is a kick count?

Your care provider may ask you to take note of the number of movements your baby makes over a two-hour period each day. Take a rest and drink a glass of juice to get her going, then keep count: your care provider will let you know roughly how many kicks you should feel.

DIARY DATES: ....

....

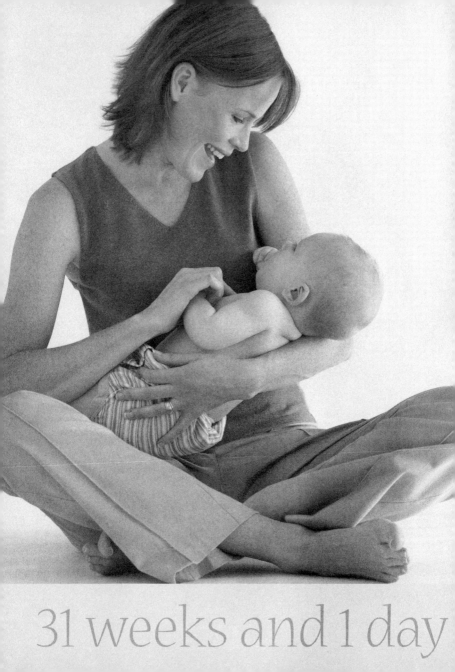

31 weeks and 1 day

62 days to go…

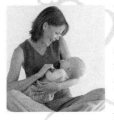

Did You Know?

If babies regularly hear the same music or stories before they are born, they recognize them immediately after birth. Babies need input in order to learn. Right from the moment of birth you must try to talk to your baby, describing what you are doing and communicating with him directly when you change or bath him. This will encourage him to experiment with sound and build up his vocabulary: by the time he is six months old he may recognize about 200 words.

Thoughts and Feelings…

....
....
....
....
....
....
....
....
....

Question

My newborn seems to sleep all the time. Is this OK?

Newborn babies tend to sleep and doze up to 18 hours a day. They often sleep in four-hour cycles—sometimes shorter. This means a new baby will wake several times during the night to be fed. They need these frequent feeds as they have such tiny stomachs.

DIARY DATES: ....
....

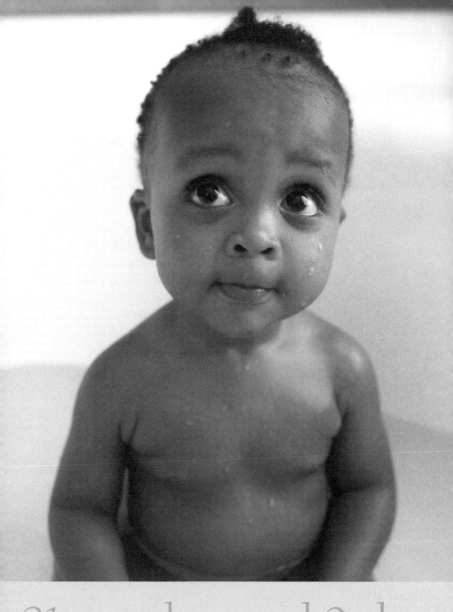

31 weeks and 2 days

61 days to go...

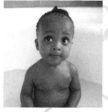

Giving Birth

The pushing phase can last anything from a few minutes up to an hour and occasionally up to two hours for a first baby. With women who have already had a child, the baby is likely to come more quickly. Contractions come less frequently and the pain of pushing changes from the intense gripping experienced during dilation to more of a burning or stinging sensation.

fact

The baby's head will first be visible at the peak of a push as a small patch of skin at the vaginal opening. The head may then recede as you rest between pushes. Finally, the baby's head crowns— or bulges out of the vagina—before she slides out: usually face down.

Thoughts and Feelings...

....
....
....
....
....
....
....
....
....
....

DIARY DATES: ....
....

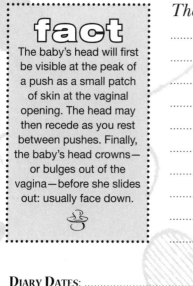

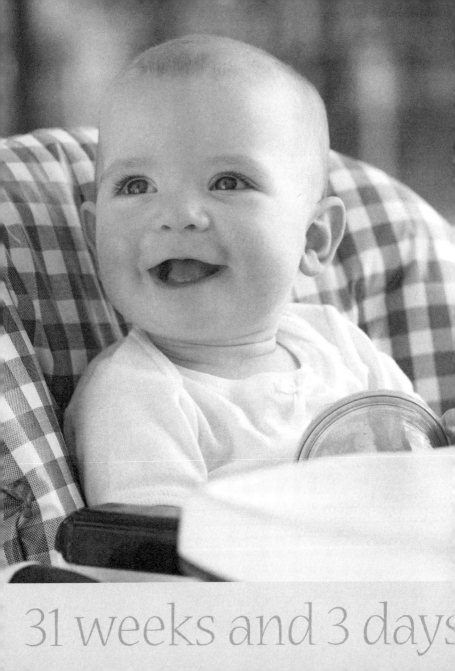

31 weeks and 3 days

60 days to go...

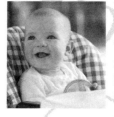

Health and Fitness

You may be experiencing the pregnancy itch. This usually takes place over your bump and may be accompanied by a rash. Calamine lotion can help. Sweating increases the itch, so wear loose clothes when possible. A lukewarm or cold shower may also help, but avoid drying yourself briskly as this can make the itch worse again. After the pregnancy this itch will simply disappear.

Thoughts and Feelings...

....

....

....

....

....

....

....

....

....

WARNING

SEVERE ITCHING IN THE LAST THREE MONTHS OF PREGNANCY, PARTICULARLY ON THE HANDS AND FEET, COULD BE AN INDICATION OF A RARE, BUT DANGEROUS LIVER DISORDER CALLED CHOLESTASIS. IF YOU ARE CONCERNED, CONSULT YOUR DOCTOR IMMEDIATELY.

DIARY DATES: ....

....

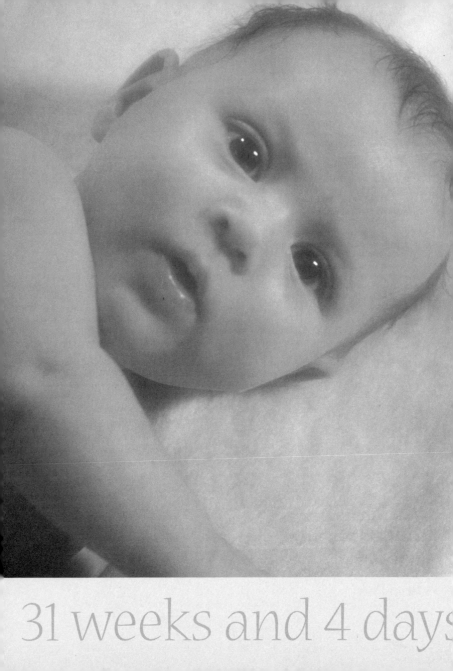

31 weeks and 4 days

59 days to go...

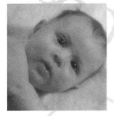

Baby's Development

The baby is actually already fully formed and the body proportions are now as you would expect them to be at birth—the body size has caught up with the head. Even though it may feel like he is being extremely active—in his confined living quarters—he is probably sleeping for 90–95% of the day. Baby is now 15¾in (40cm) long.

Thoughts and Feelings...

....

....

....

....

....

....

....

....

....

fact

Newborn babies often have slightly misshapen heads: they can become pointed from the trip down the birth canal or bruised or swollen from the use of forceps. The head will round out in a few weeks. A Cesarean baby will have a perfectly round head after being lifted out of the womb.

DIARY DATES: ....

....

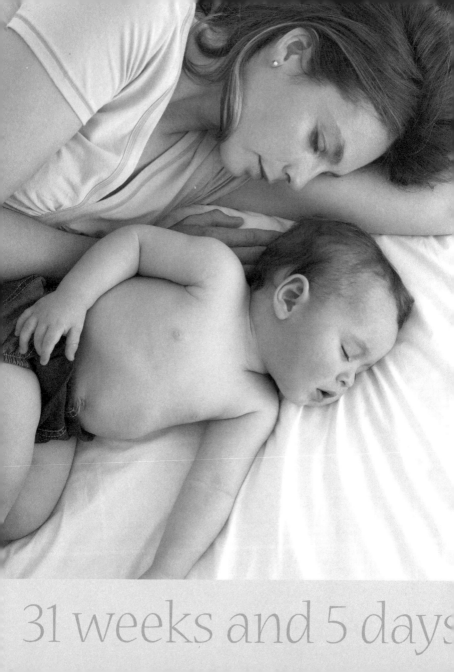
31 weeks and 5 days

58 days to go...

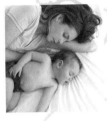

Did You Know?

Induction may be recommended if the baby is well past its due date or if you suffer from pre-eclampsia, bleeding or diabetes. Induction involves the application of prostaglandin gel to ripen your cervix for labor and delivery, and/or rupture of the membranes of the amniotic sac by your care provider. Pitocin, which stimulates contractions, may be used instead.

"If pregnancy were a book they would cut the last two chapters."

Nora Ephron, Writer

Thoughts and Feelings...

....

....

....

....

....

....

....

WARNING

INDUCTION CAN CAUSE INTENSE CONTRACTIONS AND RESULT IN A LONGER LABOR; SO CONSIDER YOUR OPTIONS CAREFULLY. MAKE SURE THE HEALTH OF YOU OR YOUR BABY IS THE MAIN REASON FOR ITS RECOMMENDATION; IT IS NOT A CHOICE TO BE MADE JUST TO TRY TO HAVE YOUR BABY AT A CONVENIENT TIME.

DIARY DATES: ....

....

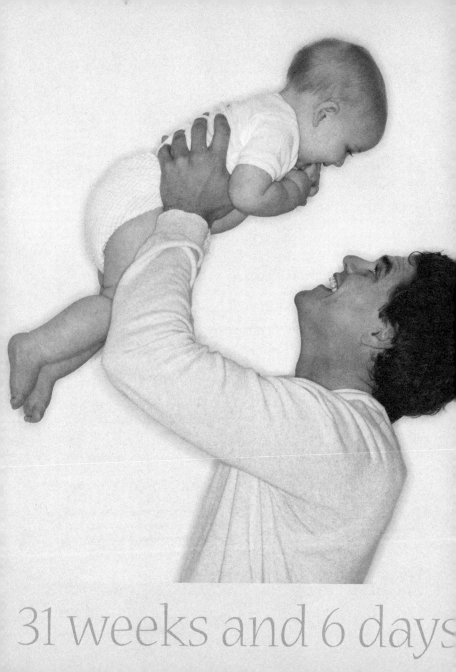

31 weeks and 6 days

57 days to go...

Baby Names for Girls and Boys

Girls
Queen (English)
Qynci (English)
Quinn (Gaelic)

Boys
Qasim (Arabic)
Quentin (Latin)
Quillan (Irish)
Quincy (French)
Quinlan (Irish)
Quinn (Irish)

Thoughts and Feelings...

....
....
....
....
....
....
....
....
....
....
....

fact

Movie stars and movie characters are a great inspiration for children's names. From Scarlett and Rhett, the central characters of the 1940s' film *Gone with the Wind* to the exotic names of today's star (Keanu, meet Uma)—the silver screen has been the inspiration for what is written on many a birth certificate.

DIARY DATES: ....
....

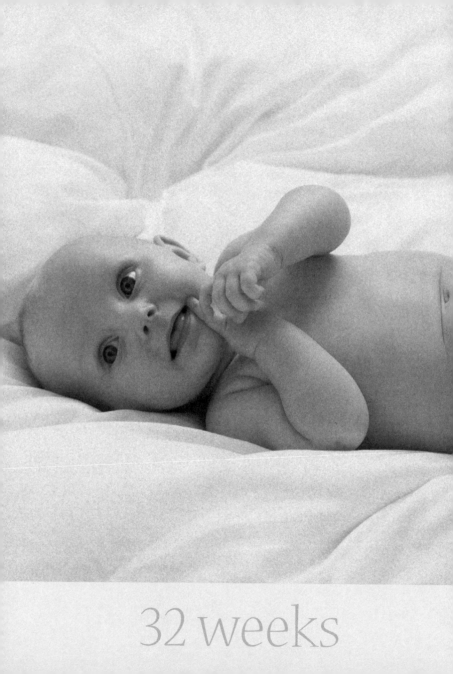

32 weeks

32 weeks

56 days to go...

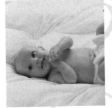

Your Pregnancy

Two more months... The moment has gradually arrived to completely finish the baby room and stock up on essentials for the first few weeks of baby's life. You will need at least four crib sheets and six light baby blankets. Even if you inherit a crib, remember that you need to buy a new mattress, as this will reduce the risk of Sudden Infant Death Syndrome.

Thoughts and Feelings...

....

....

....

....

....

....

....

....

tip · tip

WHILE YOU STILL HAVE THE ENERGY, IT MAY BE A GOOD IDEA TO FILL YOUR FREEZER. MEALS THAT YOU MAKE NOW WILL BE MEALS YOU DON'T HAVE TO WORRY ABOUT MAKING AFTER YOU HAVE BEEN UP HALF THE NIGHT FEEDING OR COMFORTING A NEW BABY.

DIARY DATES: *Check-up between weeks 32 and 34*

....

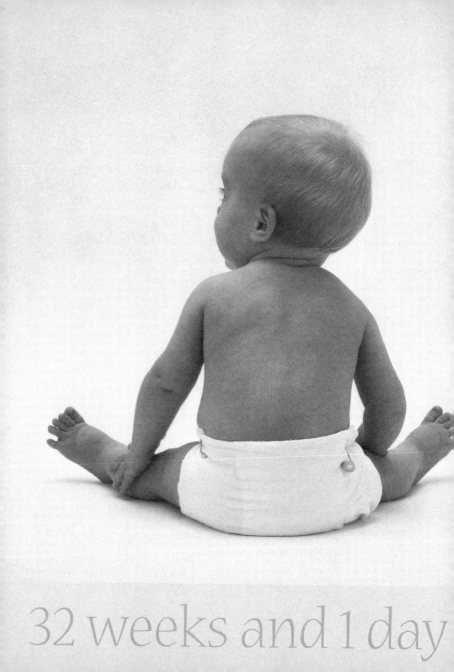

32 weeks and 1 day

55 days to go...

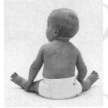

Did You Know?

Fontanelles are boneless spots between the skull plates of the baby's head. The baby has four fontanelles, the largest is on top of the head (anterior fontanelle) and can take up to 18 months to close. The other three fuse within the first four months. During delivery, the fontanelles allow the skull plates to slide towards each other, so that the head can adapt to the birth canal.

WARNING

THE FONTANELLES SHOULD NEVER BE SWOLLEN OR SUNKEN. A SUNKEN SOFT SPOT CAN INDICATE DEHYDRATION AND BULGING COULD INDICATE PRESSURE IN THE BRAIN. A NORMAL FONTANELLE SHOULD BE SLIGHTLY CURVED IN AND SOFT, YET FIRM TO THE TOUCH. CALL THE DOCTOR IMMEDIATELY IF YOU ARE WORRIED.

Thoughts and Feelings...

....

....

....

....

....

....

....

....

DIARY DATES: ....

....

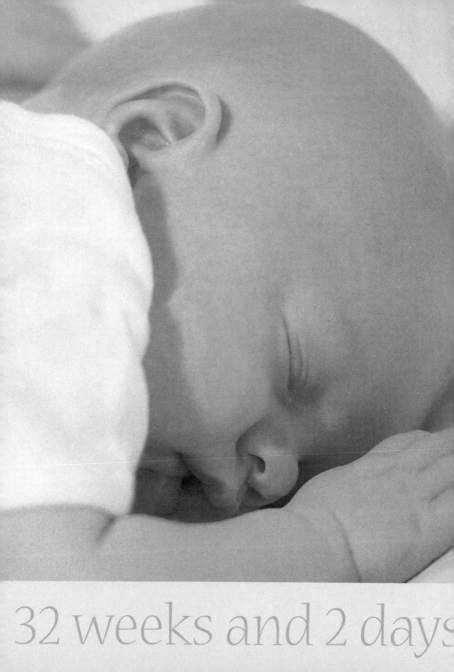

32 weeks and 2 days

54 days to go…

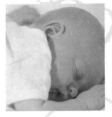

Giving Birth

After the birth of the baby you still need to push out the placenta: this is the third phase of labor. Even after baby and placenta arrive you will be monitored for at least two hours, because if the uterus fails to contract again it can lead to postpartum haemorrhage and a dive in blood pressure. If you are giving birth to multiples, you will have to wait and see what comes after your first baby: the placenta or your second child.

Thoughts and Feelings…

....

....

....

....

....

....

....

....

....

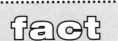

If you suffer from postpartum haemorrhage your care provider will try massage of the uterus and/or drugs to stop the bleeding, and any tear in your cervix will have to be stitched. If bleeding continues, surgery may be necessary.

DIARY DATES: ....

....

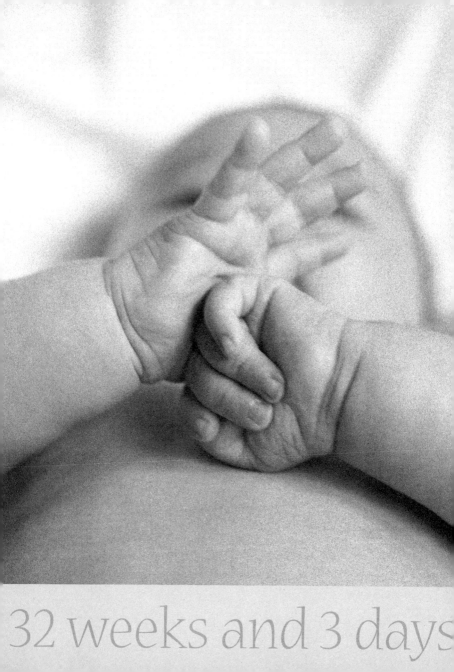

32 weeks and 3 days

53 days to go…

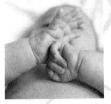

Health and Fitness

Postpartum, or post-natal, depression is a severe condition that affects 10% of new mothers. If you are worrying excessively about your new baby, or alternatively having real problems bonding with him, along with feelings of sadness, low self-esteem, decreased appetite and a lack of concentration then you should talk to your doctor. Your baby will suffer because of your anxiety and there are drugs that can help.

Thoughts and Feelings…

....
....
....
....
....
....
....
....

> **reminder**
>
> The majority of new mothers suffer from the 'baby blues'—where hormones, tiredness and dealing with a completely new experience will leave you feeling deflated and quite often tearful. This usually only lasts a few days, and you should recover quite naturally.

DIARY DATES: ....

....

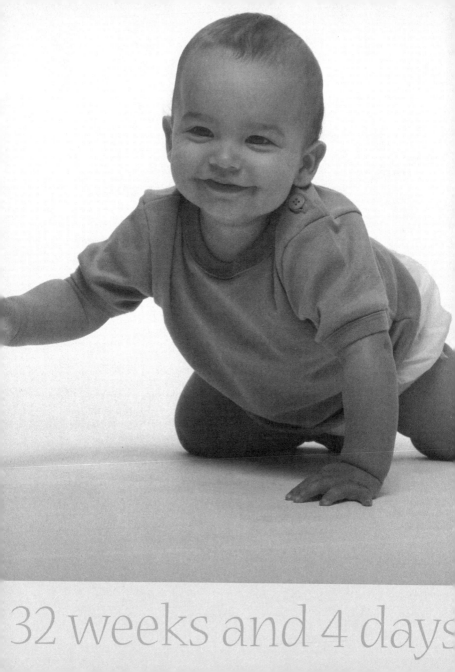

32 weeks and 4 days

52 days to go...

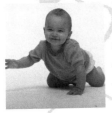

Baby's Development

The bones are becoming longer and stronger. The baby is swallowing lots of amniotic fluid and has to pass urine often. As your baby gets bigger and the space she has to move in becomes more constrained, you will have the wonderful experience of seeing tiny hands, feet and elbows—and even the occasional bottom—protruding from your belly. Your baby weighs around 4½lb (2kg) and is roughly 16½in (41cm) in length.

Thoughts and Feelings...

....

....

....

....

....

....

....

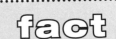

Many newborns have skin blemishes. Salmon patches or stork bites are red marks on eyelids, forehead and the nape of the neck. They will usually fade and disappear with time. Strawberry marks may at first increase in size but will usually be gone by the time the child is five.

DIARY DATES: ....

....

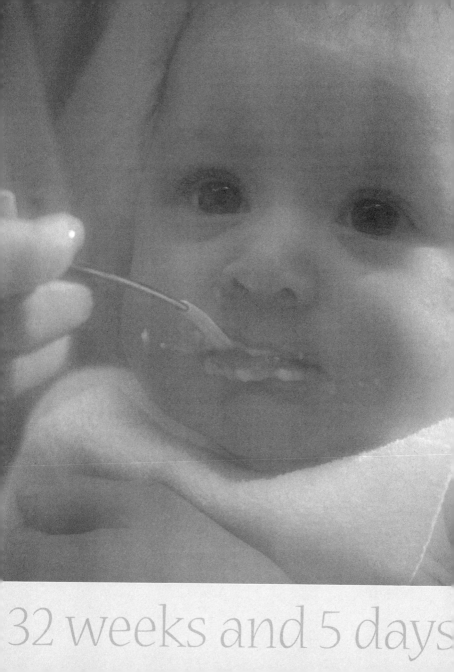

32 weeks and 5 days

51 days to go...

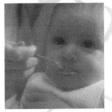

Did You Know?

'Nesting' is a common experience for expectant moms in the run-up to the due date. You may have a sudden urge to make the house perfect for your new arrival: paint the nursery, spring-clean the house, stock up on a hundred diapers. This is an instinctive need to create a safe environment for your baby: you may find you get a burst of energy that allows you to achieve all you want.

"How can there be too many children? That is like saying there are too many flowers."

Mother Teresa of Calcutta (1910–1997)

Thoughts and Feelings...

....

....

....

....

....

....

....

reminder

Your preschool child may show little interest in their new sibling. This isn't necessarily an indication of jealousy. As parents, we often want to protect our children from 'negative' feelings, but all feelings are an important part of their developing personality.

DIARY DATES: ....

....

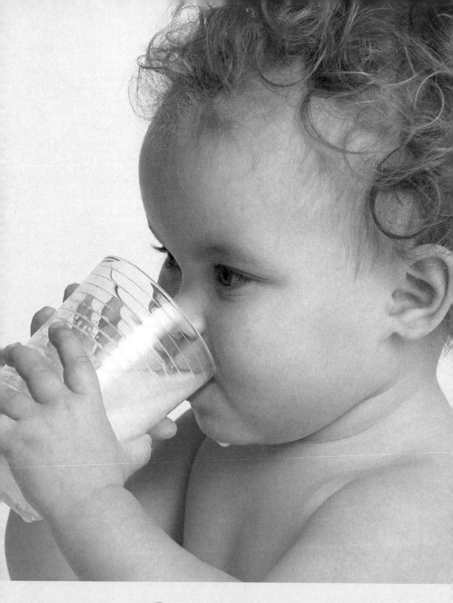

32 weeks and 6 days

50 days to go...

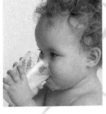

Baby Names for Girls

Rachel (Hebrew)
Ramona (Hindu)
Rebecca (Hebrew)
Rhoda (Greek)
Rhonda (Welsh)
Rita (English)

Rosamond (German)
Rosanna (English)
Rose (Latin)
Rosemary (Latin)
Ruby (English)
Ruth (Hebrew)

Thoughts and Feelings...

....
....
....
....
....
....
....
....
....
....
....

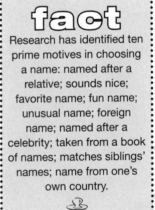

fact

Research has identified ten prime motives in choosing a name: named after a relative; sounds nice; favorite name; fun name; unusual name; foreign name; named after a celebrity; taken from a book of names; matches siblings' names; name from one's own country.

DIARY DATES: ....
....

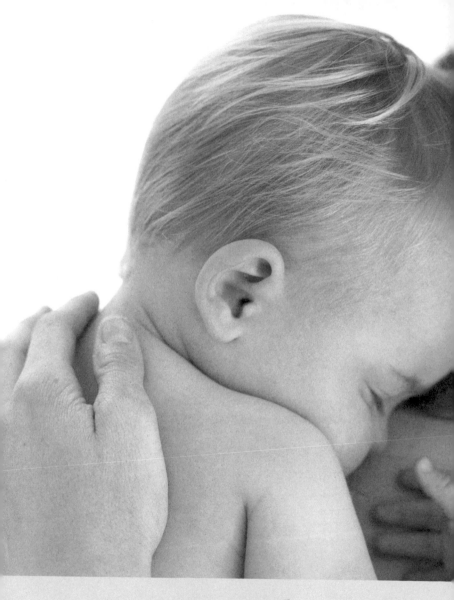

33 weeks

33 weeks

49 days to go...

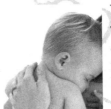

Your Pregnancy

The physical burden that pregnancy places on your body is demonstrated by your increased heartbeat. Last month your heart was making 12 extra beats a minute and this month it has increased to 15 extra beats every minute. Very high blood pressure together with water retention may sometimes indicate pre-eclampsia: this is why your blood pressure will be taken regularly in the late stages of pregnancy.

Thoughts and Feelings...

....
....
....
....
....
....
....
....
....

Question

My first sexual experience after childbirth was painful. Is this normal?

Even if you give yourself plenty of time to recover from the physical scars of childbirth, your first sexual encounter can be anything from uncomfortable to painful. Use plenty of lubrication, go gently and make sure your partner knows how it feels.

DIARY DATES: ....
....

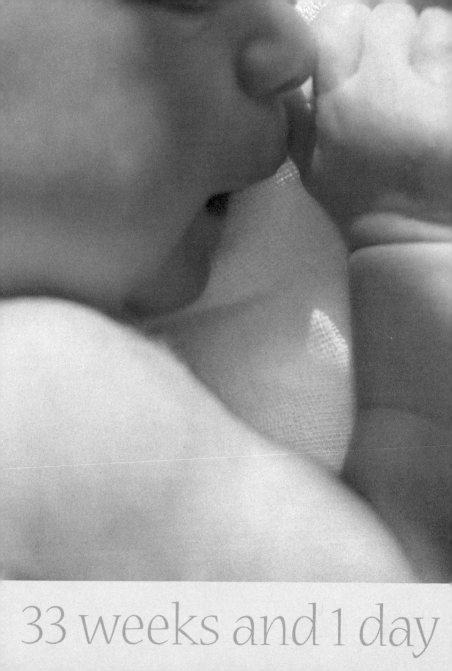

33 weeks and 1 day

48 days to go...

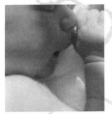

Did You Know?

A seven-week-old embryo is already moving: these are automatic movements caused by the central nervous system. You won't be aware of any of these movements and probably won't be conscious of the acrobatics until somewhere between 16 and 24 weeks. The experience of first feeling the baby move has been described as feeling like an air bubble moving around inside your stomach.

Thoughts and Feelings...

....

....

....

....

....

....

....

....

....

remember

Your toddler may feel seriously put out by the arrival of a sibling. Clinging, crying, whining, bed wetting and wakefulness are all signs of regressive toddler behaviour. Try to be patient, and not reward or punish this behavior and with time it will pass.

DIARY DATES: ....

....

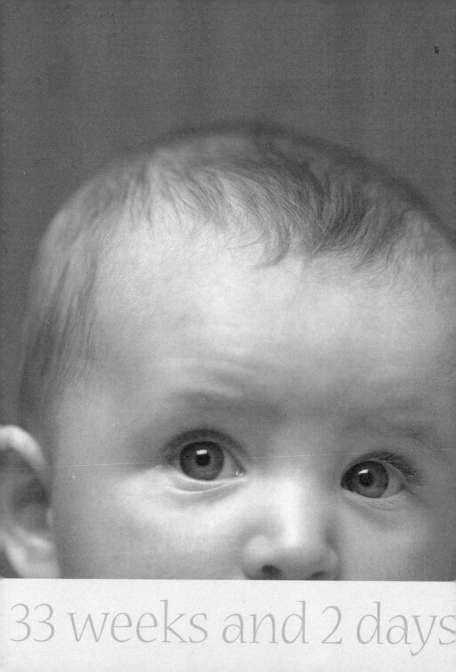

33 weeks and 2 days

47 days to go...

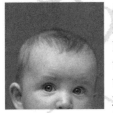

Giving Birth

Sometimes when you're pushing you'll feel like nothing is happening, that it's not going to work. Many women cannot feel clearly which way to push. If this is your first baby you will have to overcome the resistance from the bottom of the pelvis, which takes a great deal of power and time. Don't be discouraged. Pushing may cause a painful, burning feeling, but the only thing to do is to push through the pain.

fact

Little whiteheads called milia and red to purple pinpoints called petechia, are commonly found on the face of a newborn baby. Both should disappear within the first few days after birth.

Thoughts and Feelings...

....

....

....

....

....

....

....

....

....

DIARY DATES: ....

....

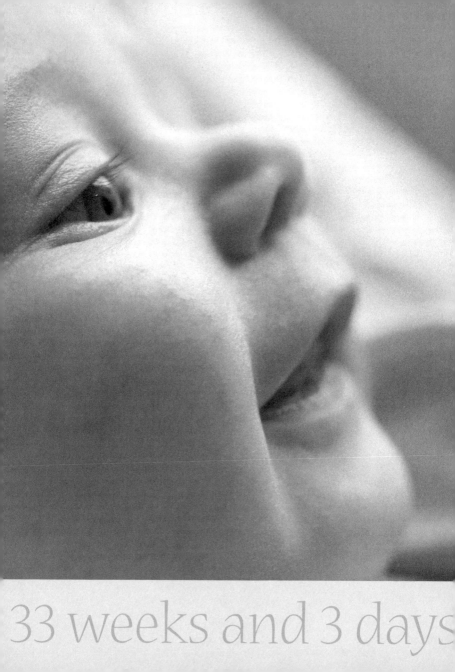

33 weeks and 3 days

46 days to go...

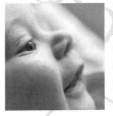

Health and Fitness

An uncommon, but nasty, after-effect of an epidural is an extreme headache brought on by a change in spinal fluid pressure if some spinal fluid should leak out into the space where the epidural is inserted. Rest and fluids usually resolve the condition, but sometimes an injection of blood into the epidural space, called a blood patch, will be required.

Thoughts and Feelings...

....

....

....

....

....

....

....

....

....

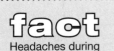

fact

Headaches during pregnancy are often related to uncertainty and fear. Anemia or the change in hormone levels can also cause headaches. If you repeatedly suffer from headaches consult your doctor or care provider.

DIARY DATES: ....

....

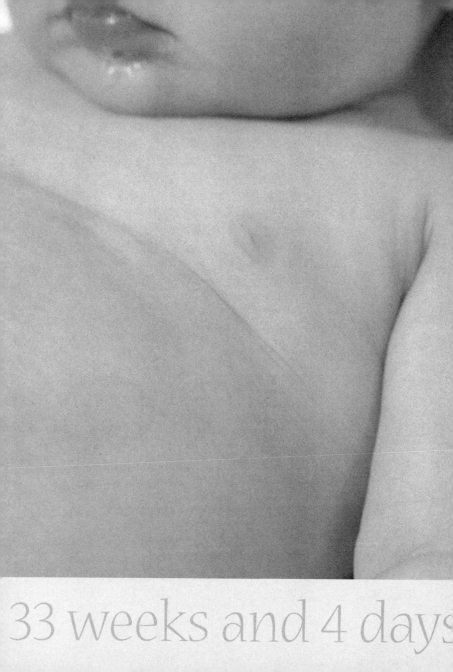

33 weeks and 4 days

45 days to go...

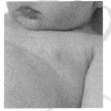

Baby's Development

The baby uses this period of the pregnancy mainly to grow and become fatter. If the mother is on the move a lot during the day and the womb is tight, the activities will often rock the baby to sleep. At night the baby will then become more active again. Crucially, the lungs are almost fully developed and the baby will be practising breathing. Baby is 16¾in (42.5cm) in length.

Thoughts and Feelings...

....

....

....

....

....

....

....

....

....

....

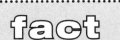

Asian and Afro-Caribbean babies are susceptible to what is known as Mongolian spots on the buttocks or lower back. They will fade over time. If your child has a bright red or purple mark, known as a port wine stain, talk to your doctor about what plastic surgery options later in life.

DIARY DATES: ....

....

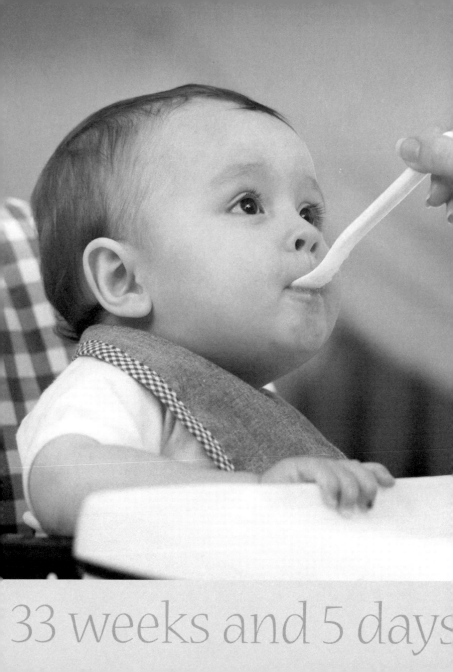

33 weeks and 5 days

44 days to go...

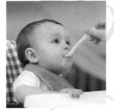

Did You Know?

The blood from the umbilical cord contains stem cells that can be crucial in treating some diseases and conditions. It is possible to collect blood from the umbilical cord then 'bank' it in a cryogenically frozen condition at a special facility, in case it is ever needed by your child in later life. However, this is a costly exercise involving an annual fee for storage, and currently it is rarely practised.

"Children are the only form of immortality we can be sure of."

Peter Ustinov, actor and playwright (1921–2004)

Thoughts and Feelings...

....

....

....

....

....

....

....

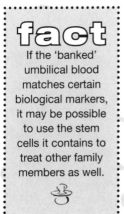

fact

If the 'banked' umbilical blood matches certain biological markers, it may be possible to use the stem cells it contains to treat other family members as well.

DIARY DATES: ....

....

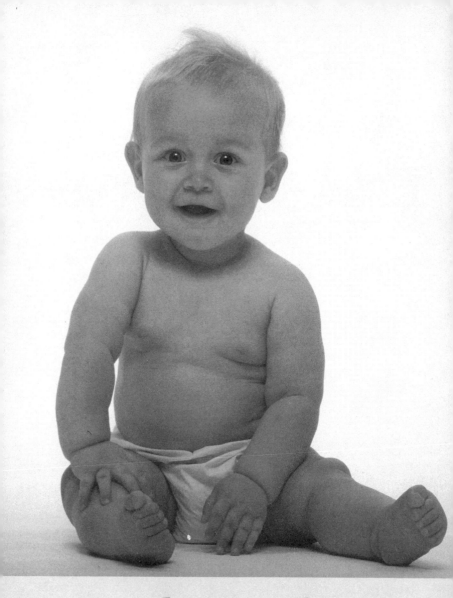

33 weeks and 6 days

43 days to go...

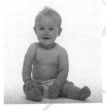

Baby Names for Boys

Ralph (English)
Raphael (Hebrew)
Raymond (German)
Reuben (Hebrew)
Richard (German)
Riley (Irish)

Robert (English)
Roger (German)
Ronald (English)
Roy (Irish)
Rupert (German)
Ryan (Irish)

Thoughts and Feelings...

....
....
....
....
....
....
....
....
....
....
....

tip · tip ·

PEOPLE HOLD SUPERSTITIONS ABOUT PARTICULAR NAMES FOR THE MOST DIVERSE OF REASONS. IF YOUR PARTNER IS DETERMINED AGAINST A NAME BECAUSE THEY ASSOCIATE IT WITH BAD LUCK OR ILLNESS, YOU MAY JUST HAVE TO DECIDE TO LET THAT NAME GO.

DIARY DATES: ....

....

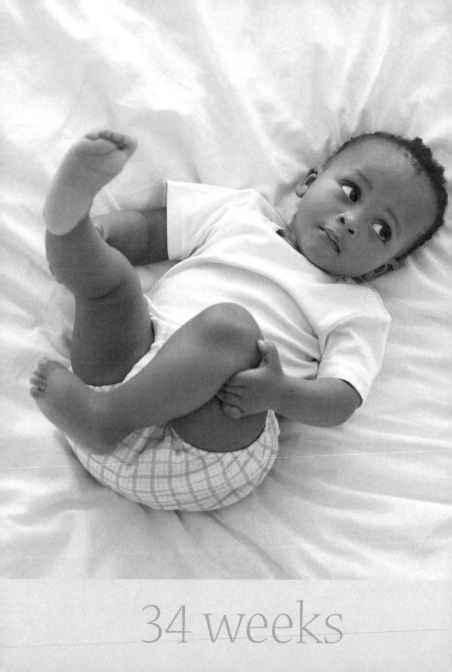

34 weeks

42 days to go...

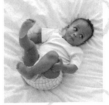

Your Pregnancy

As you get larger, towards the end of your pregnancy, you will feel increasingly uncomfortable. The baby's head may be pressing on nerves causing pain in your groin or down the inside of your legs. As the uterus expands yet more it may push the ribs up. These pains are not serious, just uncomfortable. However, if you get severe pain in your abdomen or pain with vaginal bleeding, consult your doctor immediately.

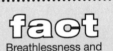

Breathlessness and increasing size will make getting around increasingly difficult. This may make you feel irritable and impatient, especially with your partner. Try to explain how you are feeling, so that he understands your mood swings.

Thoughts and Feelings...

....

....

....

....

....

....

....

....

....

DIARY DATES: ....

....

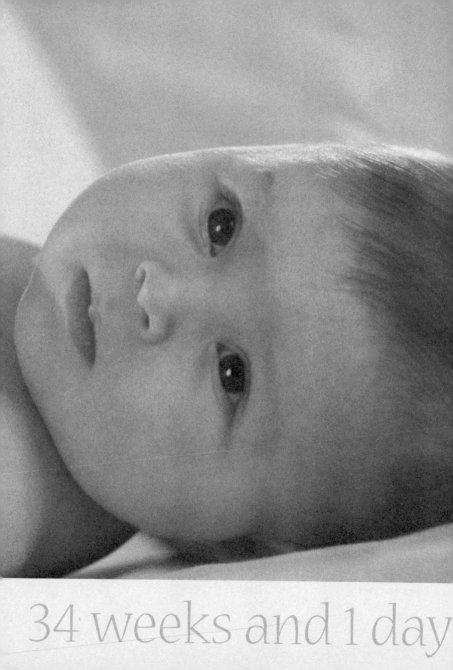

34 weeks and 1 day

41 days to go...

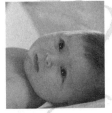

Did You Know?

Baby's first medical check-up, the Apgar test, happens just one minute after birth and again five minutes later. The Apgar is a measure of appearance, pulse, grimace (reflexes), activity and respiration. The baby is given a score of 0–2 for each category and then they are added together for a final figure: 7–10 is an average score. After this your baby will be weighed and measured and have prints taken of his feet and hands.

Thoughts and Feelings...

....

....

....

....

....

....

....

....

....

fact

For the first two months of pregnancy the baby is called an embryo. In the next four months he is called a fetus and the focus is on development. In the last three months he becomes your baby and the emphasis is on growth.

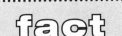

DIARY DATES: ....

....

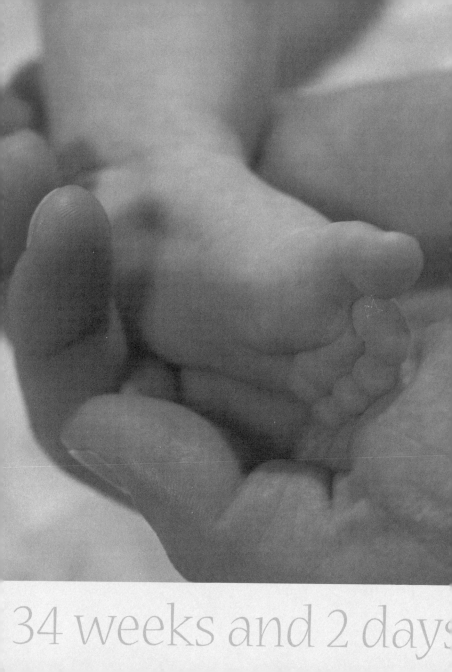

34 weeks and 2 days

40 days to go...

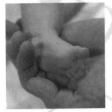

Giving Birth

Immediately after birth the umbilical cord will continue to pulse with blood for a few minutes: exactly when the cord should be cut is a matter of debate. Some care providers prefer to wait until the blood stops pulsing—or even until the placenta has been delivered—believing this is better for baby's blood pressure and reduces the mother's chances of hemorrhaging. Others think it is better to cut earlier to reduce the risk of jaundice in the baby.

Thoughts and Feelings...

....
....
....
....
....
....
....
....

Question

What if the father is unsure if he wants to cut the umbilical cord?

Many doctors will offer dad the opportunity to cut the cord. However, if you are squeamish just say no: better to get to know your new baby than spend time recovering after a fainting spell.

DIARY DATES: ....

....

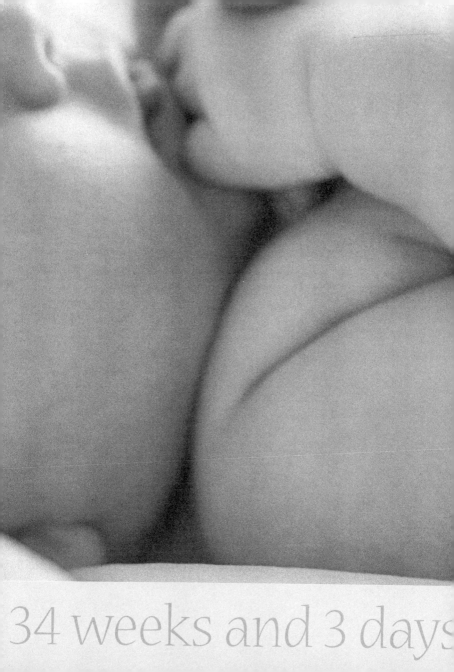

34 weeks and 3 days

39 days to go...

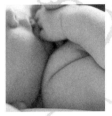

Health and Fitness

Try this breathing exercise: lie on your back with your head on a pillow and your knees bent. Place your hands on your stomach and let your legs fall out to the sides. Close your eyes and breathe in deeply through your nose, then breathe out slowly and deeply through your barely open mouth. Repeat this six times. As you breathe, imagine you are in the dilation phase and you are breathing through a contraction.

Thoughts and Feelings...

....

....

....

....

....

....

....

....

....

reminder

Continue your pelvic floor exercises after childbirth, this will firm the muscles in the pelvic floor and help to tighten your vagina after the rigors of childbirth. If you are not sure you're doing it right, practise occasionally while urinating.

DIARY DATES: ....

....

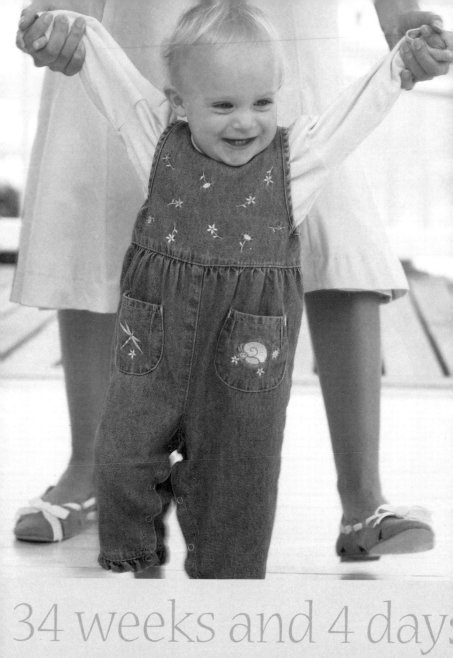

34 weeks and 4 day

38 days to go...

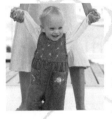

Baby's Development

The first hair (down) and the vernix, the white layer of fat protecting the baby from the liquid it lives in, are starting to flake off. Some of the vernix will remain on the baby at birth: you will see more on a baby born before its due date and less on a baby that has gone past the due date. Baby is now $17\frac{1}{8}$in (43.5cm) in length.

fact

If your baby were born today, she would have an excellent chance of surviving outside the womb. And with the special care that is now available for preterm babies she would, in all likelihood, go on to thrive.

Thoughts and Feelings...

....

....

....

....

....

....

....

....

....

....

DIARY DATES: ....

....

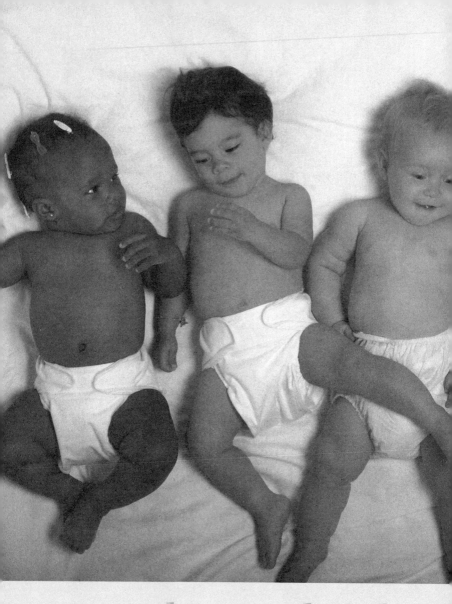

34 weeks and 5 days

37 days to go...

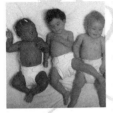

Did You Know?

For six weeks following the birth of your baby—vaginally or by Cesarean—you will be expelling lochia, a mixture of blood, mucus and tissue that comes from the site of implantation of the placenta. This will be quite heavy in the first few days after the birth and you will need extra absorbent sanitary pads. Continue to use sanitary pads; do not use tampons as they can lead to infections.

"People who say they sleep like babies usually don't have them."

Rev. Leo J Burke (1911–1980)

Thoughts and Feelings...

....

....

....

....

....

....

WARNING

IF THE LOCHIA IS SOAKING THROUGH MORE THAN ONE SANITARY PAD PER HOUR, TELL YOUR CARE PROVIDER, AS THIS COULD BE AN INDICATION THAT SOME OF THE PLACENTA HAS BEEN RETAINED IN YOUR UTERUS.

DIARY DATES: ....

....

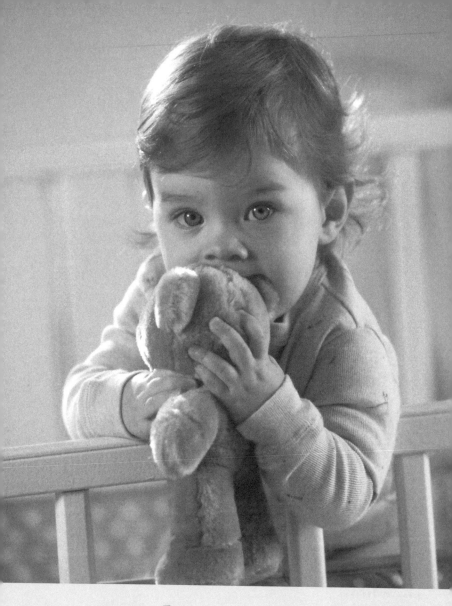

34 weeks and 6 days

36 days to go...

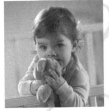

Baby Names for Girls

Sabina (Latin)
Samantha (English)
Sandra (English)
Sarah (Hebrew)
Sasha (Russian
Saskia (Dutch)

Sharon (Hebrew)
Shirley (English)
Simone (French)
Sophia (Greek)
Stephanie (French)
Susan (Hebrew)

Thoughts and Feelings...

....
....
....
....
....
....
....
....
....
....
....

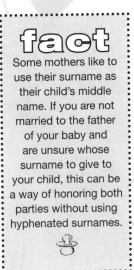

fact

Some mothers like to use their surname as their child's middle name. If you are not married to the father of your baby and are unsure whose surname to give to your child, this can be a way of honoring both parties without using hyphenated surnames.

DIARY DATES: ....
....

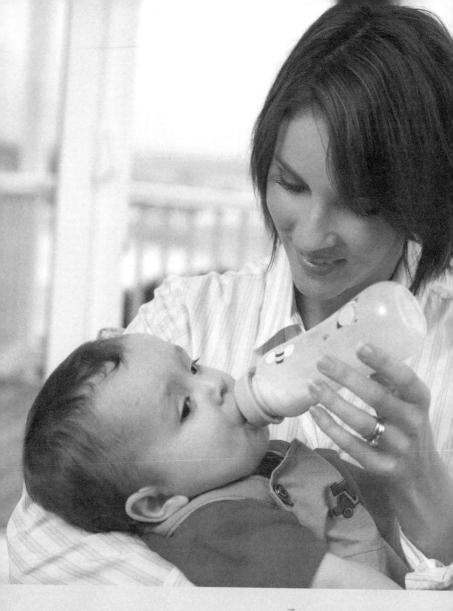

35 weeks

35 weeks

35 days to go...

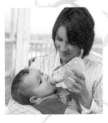

Your Pregnancy

It is time to pack your bag. You need to do this several weeks before your due date and keep it in a handy place; it is worth noting down the hospital telephone number and perhaps that of a taxi company and taping them to your bag. You need to consider three stages: first, those things you need for the labor; then, a nightgown (or two) for your hospital stay and possibly diapers and baby clothes; and, finally clothes for you and the baby to wear to go home.

Thoughts and Feelings...

....
....
....
....
....
....
....
....
....

tip · tip

IN THE FUTURE YOUR CHILD MAY BE INTERESTED IN HOW YOU FELT THROUGH YOUR PREGNANCY AND HOW THE BIRTH WENT. IT COULD BE WORTH KEEPING A DIARY OF YOUR FEELINGS AND THE DECISIONS YOU MAKE SO YOU CAN ANSWER ANY QUESTIONS IN A FEW YEARS' TIME.

DIARY DATES: ....
....

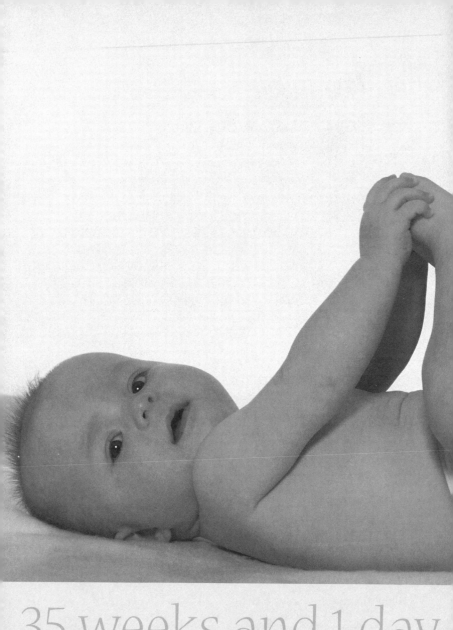

35 weeks and 1 day

34 days to go...

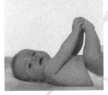

Did You Know?

An important item in your hospital bag should be your camera: it can so easily be forgotten. Don't forget batteries and film (or an extra memory card for a digital camera). Then you must make sure to actually take the photos—this, too, is sometimes forgotten in the midst of all the emotions! There'll never be another chance to record these first hours of your newborn baby's life.

Thoughts and Feelings...

....
....
....
....
....
....
....
....
....

Other essentials for your bag include a stopwatch to time contractions; personal pain relief for labor; nightgowns and a dressing gown; extra underwear; slippers; toiletries and, most importantly, your birth plan.

reminder

DIARY DATES: ....

....

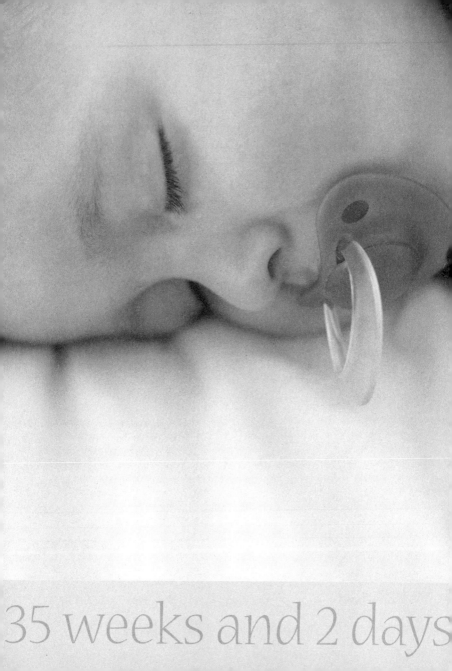

35 weeks and 2 days

33 days to go...

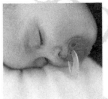

Giving Birth

In most cases, the waters do not break until your contractions are well underway. They may break spontaneously, or your care provider may pierce the membranes once dilation has progressed to a certain extent in order to check the color of the waters (amniotic fluid) and also because the water bag no longer has a function once the head has dropped properly. Your care provider may also do it to stimulate dilation if it's progressing too slowly.

Thoughts and Feelings...

....

....

....

....

....

....

....

....

tip · tip

AS YOUR DUE DATE APPROACHES YOUR PARTNER MAY WANT TO KEEP THE CAR AT LEAST HALF-FULL OF GAS AT ALL TIMES. WHEN YOU DECIDE TO GO INTO HOSPITAL HE MAY ALSO WANT TO TAKE ALONG A SNACK; AFTER ALL YOUR LABOR COULD LAST SEVERAL HOURS.

DIARY DATES: ....

....

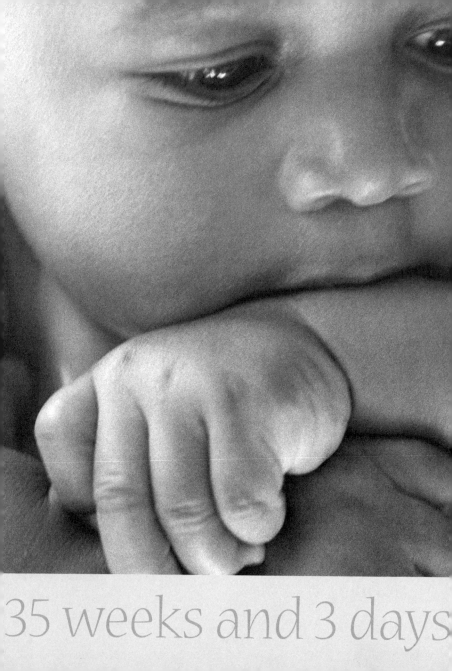

35 weeks and 3 days

32 days to go...

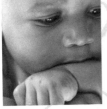

Health and Fitness

The last weeks before the birth can be both exciting and exasperating. If you are planning on working right up until delivery it is a good idea to make sure you have at least a little time to adjust to your new lifestyle, which will bring a complete change of pace. Try to build in a moment of rest before the big moment, and this will help you to start labor calmly and without fear.

Thoughts and Feelings...

....

....

....

....

....

....

....

....

....

reminder

If you are planning to return to the same job after the baby is born, you will want things to run smoothly while you are away. Get everything in order and let colleagues know whether or not you wish to be contacted at home during maternity leave.

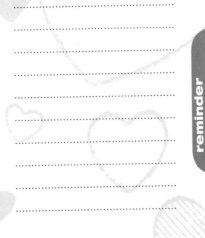

DIARY DATES: ....

....

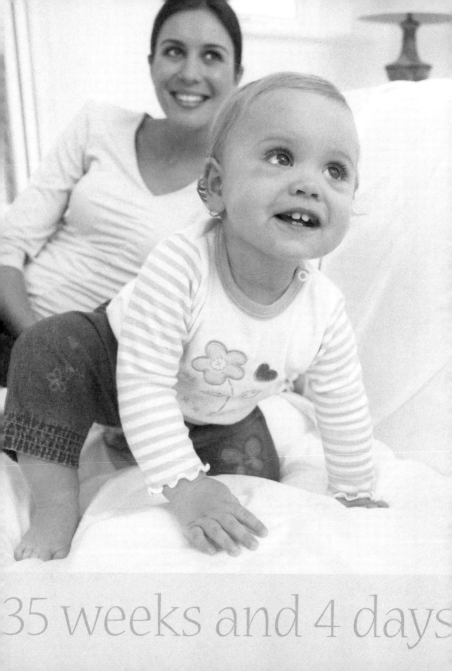

35 weeks and 4 days

31 days to go...

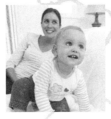

Baby's development

Over the next few weeks the baby's weight will increase by almost 1oz (30g) a day. The iris of the eyes is blue and eyebrows and eyelashes are fully grown. The nails have grown to the tips of the fingers and toes. The hair on the baby's head may very well be 1–2in (2.5–5cm) long by now. If you are having a little boy, his testicles will have descended and can be seen on a scan. Baby is about 18in (45cm) long.

Thoughts and feelings...

....
....
....
....
....
....
....
....
....

Putting on weight is the most important thing your baby can do at this late stage of the pregnancy. The average weight of a baby at birth is 7.5lb (3.4kg).

DIARY DATE: ....

....

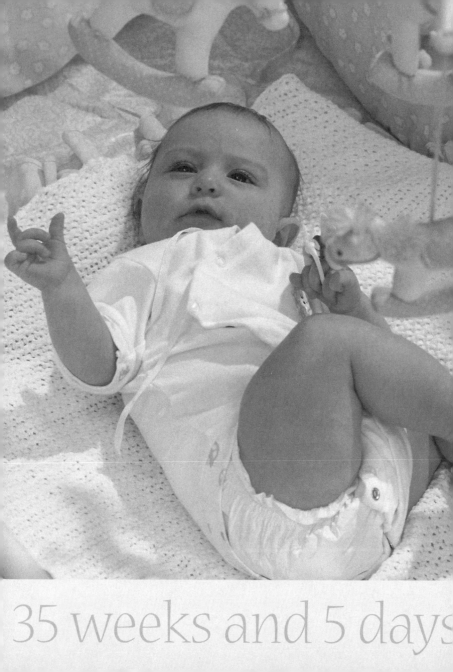

35 weeks and 5 days

30 days to go...

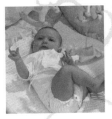

Did you know?

A breast pump is a great way to increase your supply of breast milk, or to express milk for others to feed to your baby. A manual pump is the least expensive option and is easy to transport. However, it is not hugely efficient and will take some time to empty a breast. A hospital-style electric pump is the most efficient, but also very expensive. However, it is possible to hire these pumps through your hospital or a lactation consultant or business.

"If your baby is 'beautiful and perfect, never cries or fusses, sleeps on schedule and burps on demand, an angel all the time,' you're the grandma."

Theresa Bloomingdale, author

Thoughts and feelings...

....

....

....

....

DIARY DATE: ....

....

fact

If you rent an electric breast pump you will have to purchase a personal kit for use with the unit. This comprises everything that comes in contact with your breast milk including tubing and bottles.

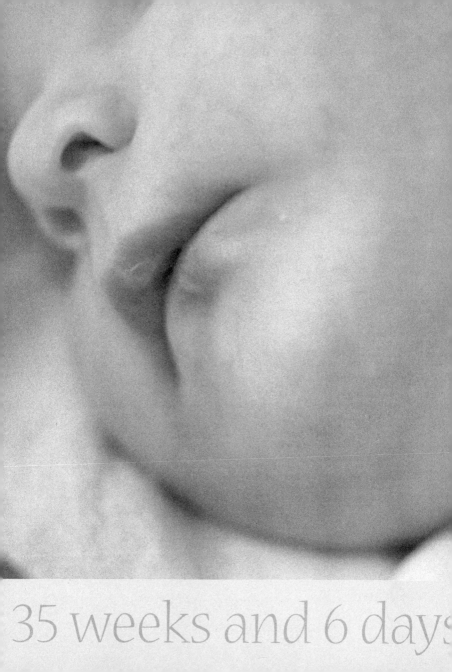

35 weeks and 6 days

29 days to go...

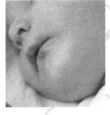

Baby names for boys

Samuel (Hebrew)   Sinclair (French)
Scott (English)   Spencer (English)
Sean (Irish)   Stanley (English)
Sebastian (Latin)   Stephen (Greek)
Seth (Hebrew)   Stewart (English)
Seymour (French)   Sylvester (Latin)
Simon (Hebrew)

Thoughts and feelings...

....
....
....
....
....
....
....
....
....
....

If you and your partner can't agree on whose surname the baby will take, you could try using a last name as a first name. Surnames such as Morgan, Windsor or even Smith can work quite well when used as a first name.

DIARY DATE: ....

....

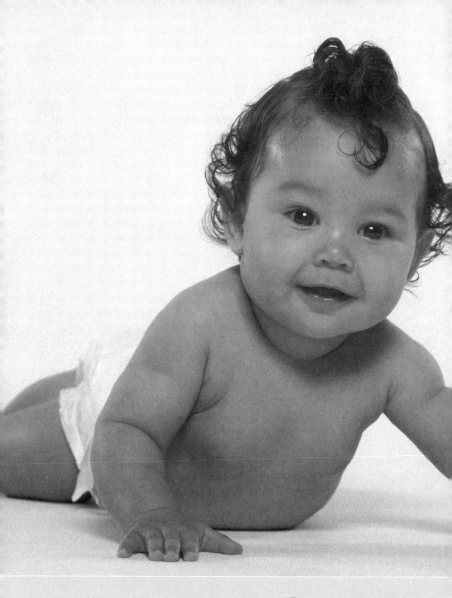

36 weeks

36 weeks

28 days to go...

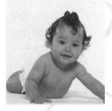

Your pregnancy

Resting should be an important part of your schedule. Working women may already have stopped, or are going to do so very soon. And rightly so! Also, don't forget that giving birth takes up a great deal of energy. It is important that you are fresh when you start. Too much exertion will immediately result in a hard stomach. This is your body telling you to take a rest now!

Thoughts and feelings...

....

....

....

....

....

....

....

....

....

fact

Breastfeeding burns about 500 calories a day but you probably only need to increase your intake by 300 calories, as your body has plenty to spare at the moment and has stored it just for this purpose. Take plenty of fluids as well—preferably water.

DIARY DATE: *Check-up between 36 and 38 weeks*

....

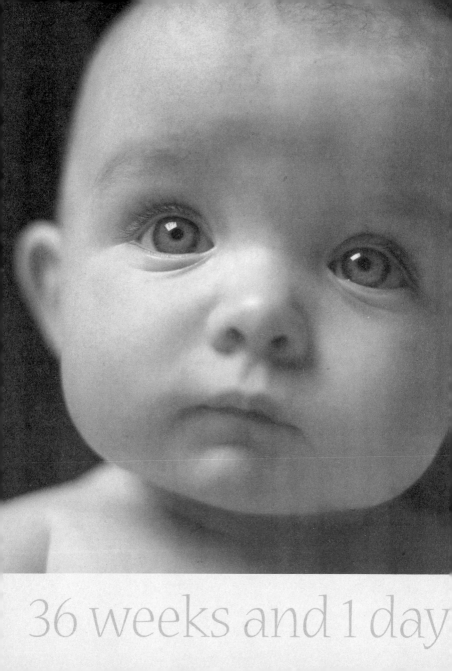

36 weeks and 1 day

27 days to go...

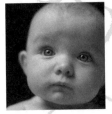

Did you know?

Mastitis is an infection caused by a blocked milk duct. Symptoms include a warm breast; red, tender streaks on the breast, pain and swelling and running a temperature. Keep breastfeeding your baby as the infection cannot harm her and it will help to ease the condition. A warm hot-water bottle, warm compresses or a hot shower can also ease pain. If it doesn't clear itself in a few days or your condition worsens, contact your doctor.

Thoughts and feelings...

....
....
....
....
....
....
....
....
....

Q&A

Can I become pregnant while breastfeeding?

The chances of becoming pregnant are reduced while breastfeeding. But even if you are breastfeeding eight to nine times a day, there's still always a 30% chance of your becoming pregnant.

DIARY DATE: ....

....

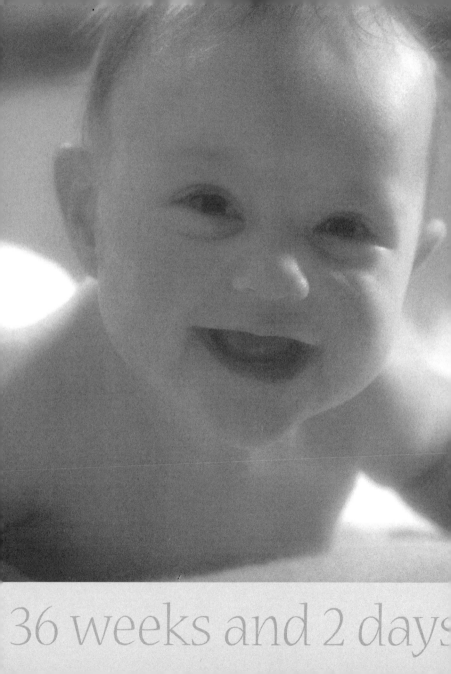

36 weeks and 2 days

26 days to go...

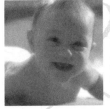

Giving birth

A woman generally loses ½–1pt (0.25–0.5L) of blood while giving birth. During pregnancy your blood volume increases substantially so you should be able to manage this. After the birth is when loss of blood can become serious if postpartum hemorrhaging occurs. This is why you will be kept in hospital for some hours after delivery and regular checkups will be made.

Thoughts and feelings...

....
....
....
....
....
....
....
....
....

fact

Giving birth, either vaginally or by Cesarean section, can be a bloody affair and your partner may not respond well to the sight of blood. It is better for him to step outside the delivery room for a minute or two rather than to sidetrack your carers to peel him off the floor should he faint.

DIARY DATE: ....
....

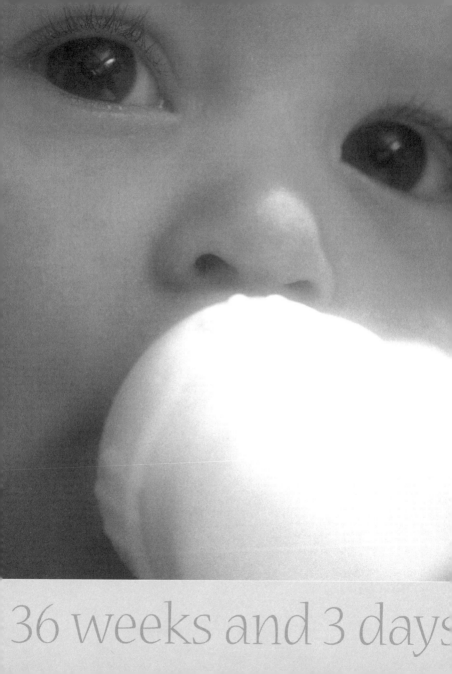
36 weeks and 3 days

25 days to go...

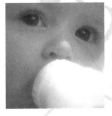

Health and fitness

In the last weeks of your pregnancy your sleep will become more and more disturbed. This may bring you to the conclusion that you will manage those sleepless nights with a new baby quite well. However, three weeks after the birth you may feel like a zombie who constantly craves sleep. Remember, sleep whenever your baby sleeps and hold onto the fact that your baby will eventually sleep through the night.

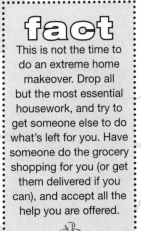

fact

This is not the time to do an extreme home makeover. Drop all but the most essential housework, and try to get someone else to do what's left for you. Have someone do the grocery shopping for you (or get them delivered if you can), and accept all the help you are offered.

Thoughts and feelings...

....

....

....

....

....

....

....

....

....

DIARY DATE: ....

....

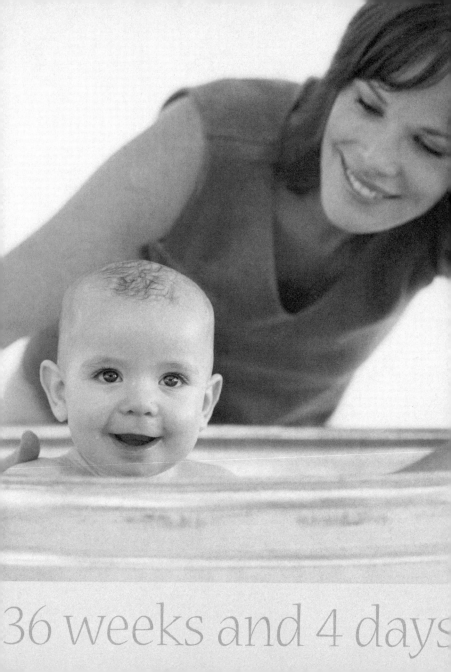

36 weeks and 4 days

24 days to go...

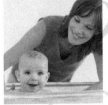

Baby's development

The baby is getting so heavy now that she will drop deeper into the pelvis. Sometimes, this is accompanied by labor pains or sharp, shooting pains. After the baby has dropped you will feel less breathless as the baby allows you more lung space. The baby will continue to practise breathing movements, even though there is no air in the lungs. Baby is roughly 18½in (46.5cm) long.

Thoughts and feelings...

....

....

....

....

....

....

....

....

....

fact

Your newborn infant may arrive in need of a manicure and pedicure. The nails that have been growing for many months now will be in need of a trim. Use sharp scissors or infant-sized clippers. It's a job best done while your baby is sleeping.

DIARY DATE: ....

....

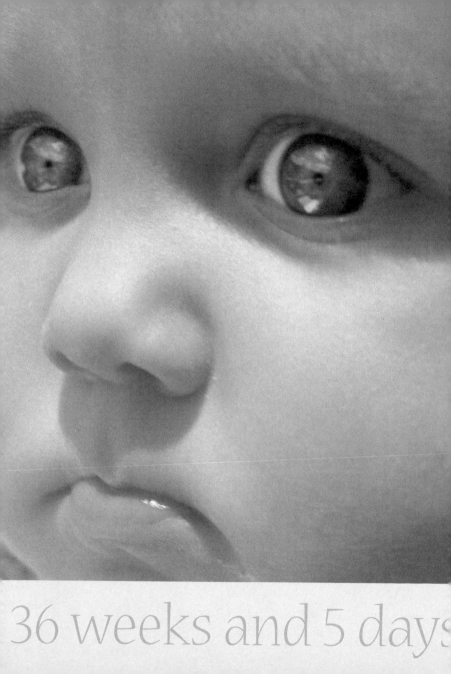

36 weeks and 5 days

23 days to go...

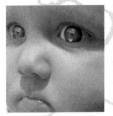

Did you know?

Premature babies who have to spend time in intensive care have been found to benefit from 'kangaroo care'—that is skin-to-skin contact with their mother. It can be emotionally draining for a new mother to see her baby attached to lots of wires, and it can be particularly distressing if you are not allowed to touch your baby. The staff are trained to take the best care of your baby and they will let you know the most important ways you can help.

> *"A baby is God's opinion that the world should go on."*
>
> **Carl Sandburg, poet (1878–1967)**

Thoughts and feelings...

....
....
....
....
....
....

tip · tip

TRY TO GET AS INVOLVED WITH THE CARE OF YOUR PREMATURE BABY AS YOU CAN; HOLDING A TINY HAND, HELPING TO FEED OR CHANGE HER WHEN YOU CAN AND UNDERSTANDING ANY SPECIAL MEDICAL NEEDS SHE MAY HAVE.

DIARY DATE: ....
....

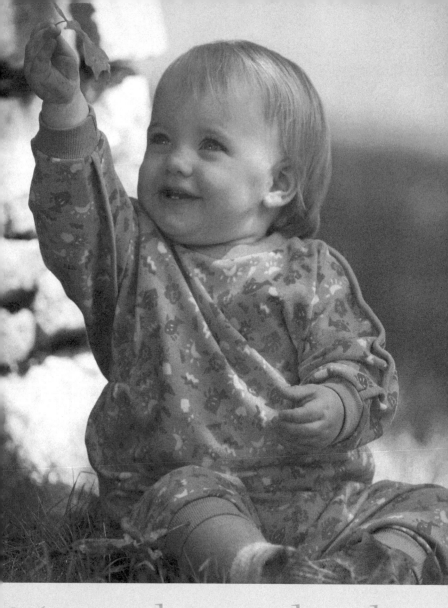

36 weeks and 6 days

22 days to go...

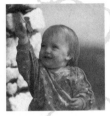

Baby names for girls

Tabitha (English)
Tamara (Hebrew)
Tatiana (Russian)
Teresa (Greek)
Tessa (Polish)

Thelma (Greek)
Theodora (Greek)
Thora (Scandinavian)
Tiffany (Greek)
Tracy (English)

Thoughts and feelings...

....
....
....
....
....
....
....
....
....
....

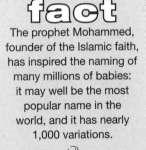

fact

The prophet Mohammed, founder of the Islamic faith, has inspired the naming of many millions of babies: it may well be the most popular name in the world, and it has nearly 1,000 variations.

DIARY DATE: ....

....

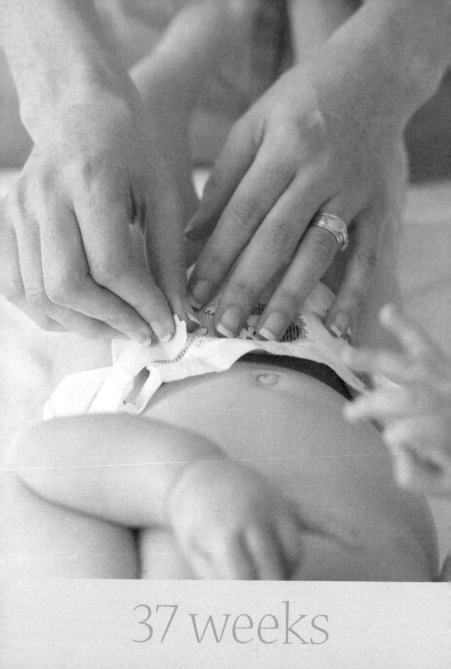

37 weeks

21 days to go...

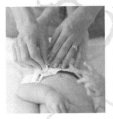

Your pregnancy

In the womb your baby gets used to all kinds of noise. Noises in the street, noises at home and noises from inside your body. If you play the same music regularly, particularly as you are relaxing, there is a good chance that once she is born your baby will find this particular piece of music calming and soothing: subconsciously, she will associate it with her safe existence in the womb.

Thoughts and feelings...

....

....

....

....

....

....

....

....

....

Q&A

My weight has actually gone down 1lb (450g) recently. Should I be worried?

In this last month, it is possible you will lose a small amount of weight. Baby continues to grow but your weight loss is due to a drop in amniotic fluid production.

DIARY DATE: ....

....

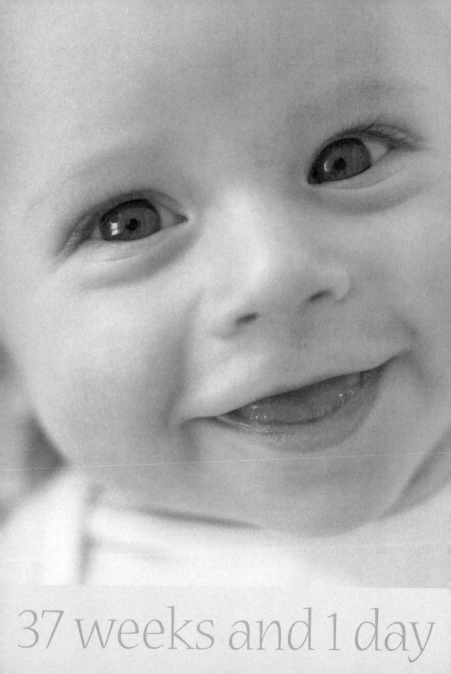

37 weeks and 1 day

20 days to go...

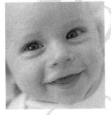

Did you know?

As the baby drops or as your pelvic joints begin to soften in preparation for delivery you may find that you are suffering from constant pain in the pubic bone, tailbone (coccyx) hips and lower back. Talk to your care provider and find out if there is a physiotherapist who specializes in prenatal care that you could see. They may be able to give you some pain relief.

Thoughts and feelings...

....
....
....
....
....
....
....
....
....
....

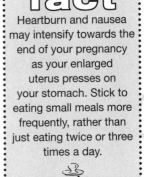

fact

Heartburn and nausea may intensify towards the end of your pregnancy as your enlarged uterus presses on your stomach. Stick to eating small meals more frequently, rather than just eating twice or three times a day.

DIARY DATE: ....
....

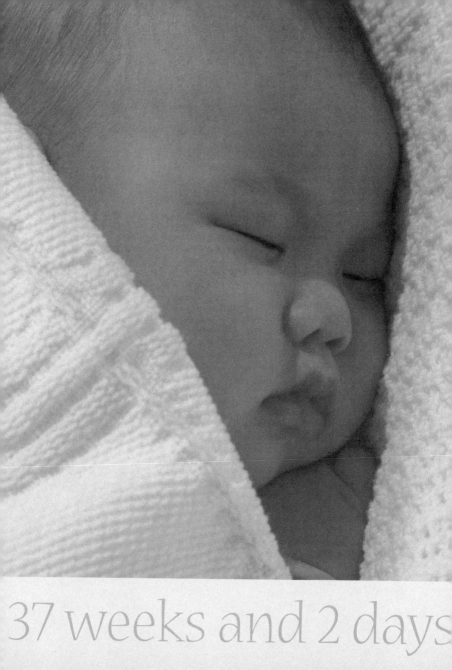

37 weeks and 2 days

19 days to go...

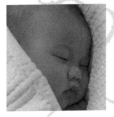

Giving birth

If you notice one or more of the following things, you can be sure you won't have to wait much longer: the mucus plug from the neck of the womb 'shows' as a small amount of bloodstained mucus; the membranes of the amniotic sac burst and you have a trickle or gush of clear liquid; you experience regular contractions that don't go away but come closer together over time.

fact

In the last weeks of pregnancy your care provider will check your cervix to see if it is preparing for the delivery. He or she will also check to see if baby has dropped towards the pelvis.

Thoughts and feelings...

....
....
....
....
....
....
....
....
....

DIARY DATE: ....
....

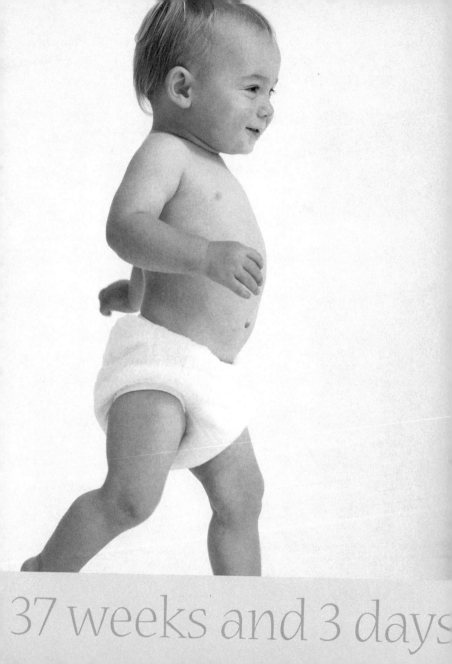

37 weeks and 3 days

18 days to go...

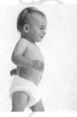

Health and fitness

The exact causes of post-natal depression are unclear. A rapid decline in hormone levels after the delivery of the placenta may be one contributing factor. You are more at risk of post-natal depression if you have a history of depression, panic attacks, obsessive-compulsive disorders, premenstrual syndrome or previous attacks of post-natal depression. Let your care provider know if you fall into any of these categories.

Thoughts and feelings...

....
....
....
....
....
....
....

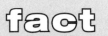

fact

If you are in an unsupportive or even abusive relationship, and feel alone with dealing with the stresses of a new baby, you are also more likely to be at risk of post-natal depression.

DIARY DATE: ....

....

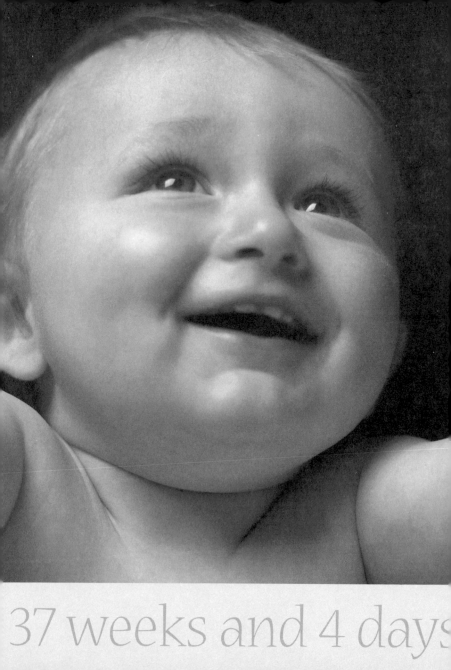

37 weeks and 4 days

17 days to go...

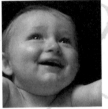

Baby's development

The baby's skin is now nice and smooth. Some of the skull bones are not yet fused: the fontanelles—areas on the baby's skull where the bones are not joined together—remain flexible to aid the baby's passage down the birth canal. The lungs, the final organ to fully mature, now has enough surfactant for the baby to breathe independently outside of the womb. The baby is 19in(48cm) in length.

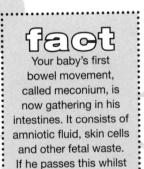

fact

Your baby's first bowel movement, called meconium, is now gathering in his intestines. It consists of amniotic fluid, skin cells and other fetal waste. If he passes this whilst still in the womb it can lead to complications.

Thoughts and feelings...

....
....
....
....
....
....
....
....
....

DIARY DATE: ....
....

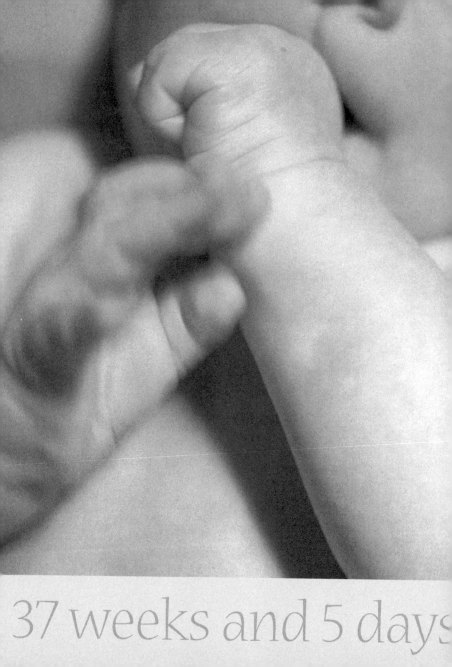

37 weeks and 5 days

16 days to go...

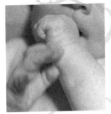

Did you know?

Stress, caused by lack of sleep and dealing with a very new experience, can lead to difficulties with breastfeeding, although the degree to which this is true varies considerably from woman to woman. Stress and fatigue can increase levels of adrenaline, which inhibit oxytocin, crucial to the letdown reflex, which can result in your baby having to work much harder to get the milk she needs.

"There never was a child so lovely but his mother was glad to get him to sleep."

Ralph Waldo Emerson, author and popular philosopher (1803–1882)

Thoughts and feelings...

....

....

....

....

....

fact

Many people, from your care provider to your relatives, will encourage you to nap when the baby is sleeping. This is good advice and is the only reasonable way to get through the first few weeks of caring for a new baby.

DIARY DATE: ....

....

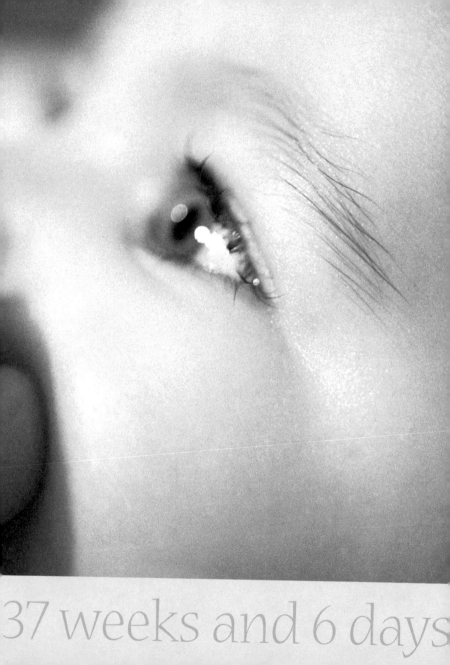

37 weeks and 6 days

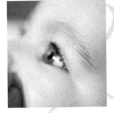

Baby names for boys

Tanner (English)
Taylor (English)
Terence (Latin)
Theodore (Greek)
Thomas (Aramaic)
Timothy (Greek)

Tobias (Hebrew)
Tony (Latin)
Travis (French)
Trevor (Welsh)
Tristan (Welsh)
Tyler (English)

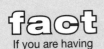

fact

If you are having multiples, twins or more, it can be tempting to choose names with a similar sound such as Tammy and Sammy. This isn't helpful for your children: as they grow they will find it hard to differentiate between the sounds and this could hinder their ability to develop their individual identity.

Thoughts and feelings...

....
....
....
....
....
....
....
....
....
....
....

DIARY DATE: ....

....

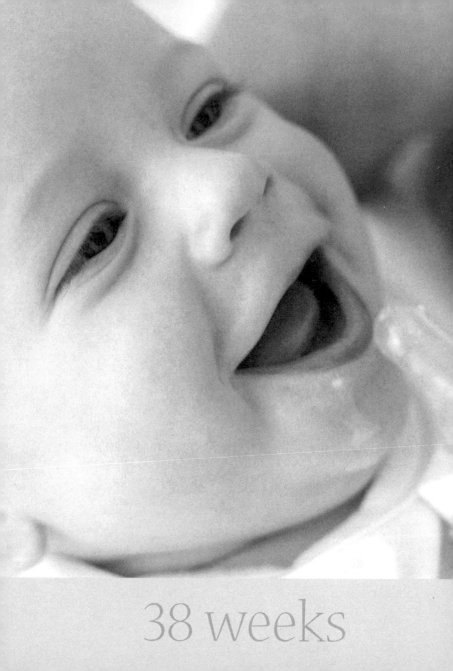

38 weeks

38 weeks

14 days to go...

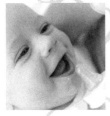

Your pregnancy

Especially during the last weeks of pregnancy, sleeping becomes increasingly difficult. In addition, you may be feeling anxious about labour and then about your new life as a mother. This may add up to irritability: try to keep away from people who trigger this irritation and leave your partner to answer the increasing number of phone calls asking if anything has happened yet.

Thoughts and feelings...

....

....

....

....

....

....

....

....

....

remember

If you have a long list of family and friends you wish to call from the hospital, your partner will need plenty of small change. Most hospitals ask you to turn off mobile phones as they can interfere with sensitive medical equipment.

DIARY DATE: ....

....

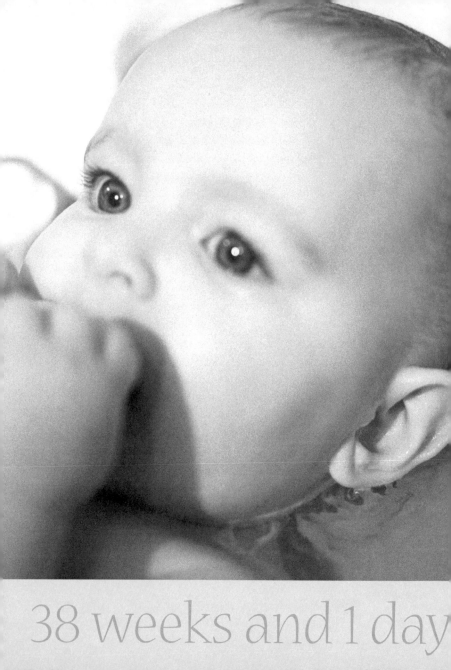

38 weeks and 1 day

13 days to go…

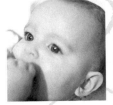

Did you know?

Your body is so adapted for breastfeeding that if you give birth prematurely you produce preterm milk that is high in fats, proteins and sugars to help your baby gain the weight he needs. After about a month, your body starts to manufacture mature milk. If your baby is full-term then mature milk is fully in place roughly five days after you give birth.

Thoughts and feelings…

....
....
....
....
....
....
....
....
....
....

remember

Your breast milk comes in two servings. From each breast your baby receives foremilk, which makes up about one-third of what she drinks, followed by hindmilk, which is rich in nutrients and fat. She needs both to thrive.

DIARY DATE: ....

....

38 weeks and 2 day

12 days to go...

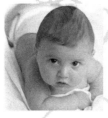

Giving birth

After an assisted birth (a forceps delivery or vacuum delivery) your baby may be placed in an incubator for observation. The rules for this will differ from one hospital to another. After a Caesarean section performed under a general anaesthetic, it is also very likely the baby will be placed in an incubator as the anaesthetic will affect him.

fact

During the first two years of his life, a premature baby will be assessed based on his due date, rather than his actual arrival date. Thus a six-month-old who came a month early will be checked for the developmental abilities of a five-month-old.

Thoughts and feelings...

....
....
....
....
....
....
....
....
....
....

DIARY DATE: ....
....

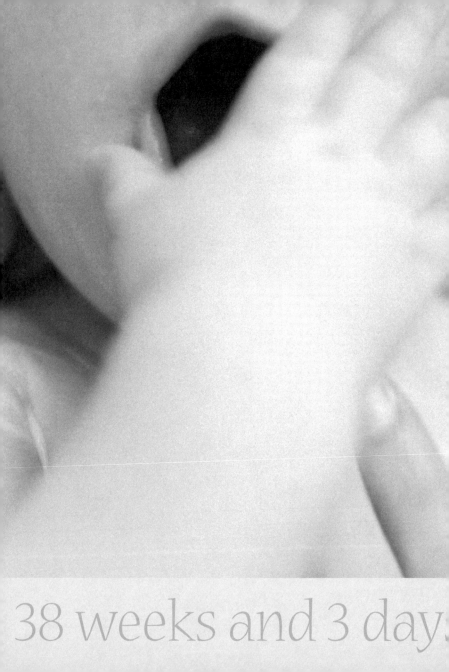

38 weeks and 3 days

11 days to go...

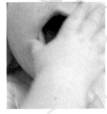

Health and fitness

If you put your tightest pre-pregnancy trousers into your bag as your coming home outfit, you are sure to be disappointed. Although you will have shed a considerable burden with the delivery of your child and the placenta, it will take several weeks for you to return to your old shape. If the idea of putting maternity clothes back on is depressing, invest in a new, loose and flexible outfit.

Thoughts and feelings...

....
....
....
....
....
....
....
....
....

remember

Eating a light, easily digestible snack such as a biscuit or toast during labour may help keep your strength up. However, many care providers will want you to keep eating to a minimum in case an emergency general anesthetic is needed.

DIARY DATE: ....

....

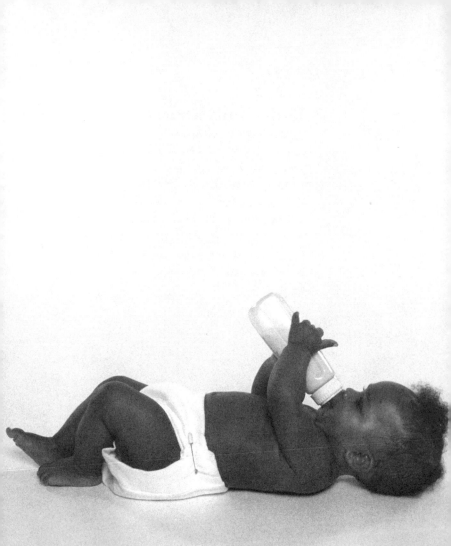

38 weeks and 4 days

10 days to go...

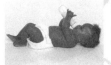

Baby's development

In these last weeks the baby is mainly building up her strength, putting on weight and growing. She is lying all folded up, often with her hands under her chin, near her ears or against her cheeks. Inside her cramped living quarters she barely has room to move and the average weight of a baby at this point is just over 6½lb (3kg). She is roughly 19½in (49cm).

Thoughts and feelings...

....

....

....

....

....

....

....

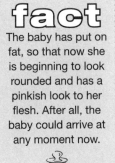

fact

The baby has put on fat, so that now she is beginning to look rounded and has a pinkish look to her flesh. After all, the baby could arrive at any moment now.

DIARY DATE: ....

....

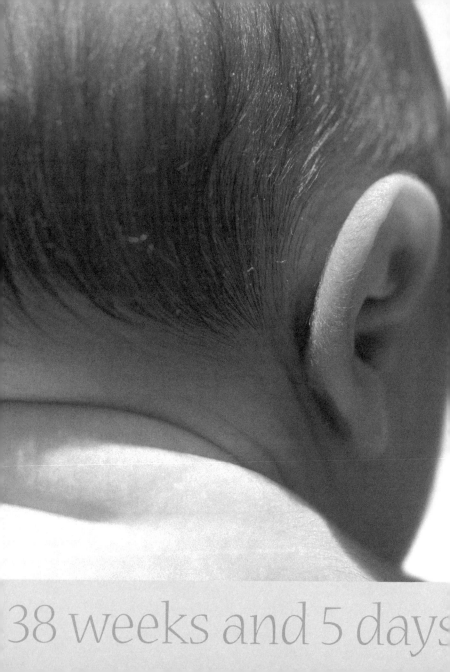

38 weeks and 5 days

9 days to go...

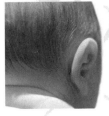

Did you know?

All babies take in air when they feed, whether by breast or bottle. They need burping after feeding to avoid air bubbles accumulating in their stomachs and causing pain. Either place your baby over your shoulder and gently rub or pat his back, or sit him on your lap supporting his chest and chin with one hand while rubbing his back with the other or lay him on his tummy across your lap and burp him.

"I have found the best way to give advice to your children is to find out what they want and then advise them to do it."

Harry S. Truman, American president (1884–1972)

Thoughts and feelings...

....

....

....

....

....

....

remember

Make your feeding station as comfortable as possible. Choose a chair with plenty of support and use pillows as well. Have a table close by with light for reading by. If you are breastfeeding, you will need a glass of water as you are bound to get thirsty.

DIARY DATE: ....

....

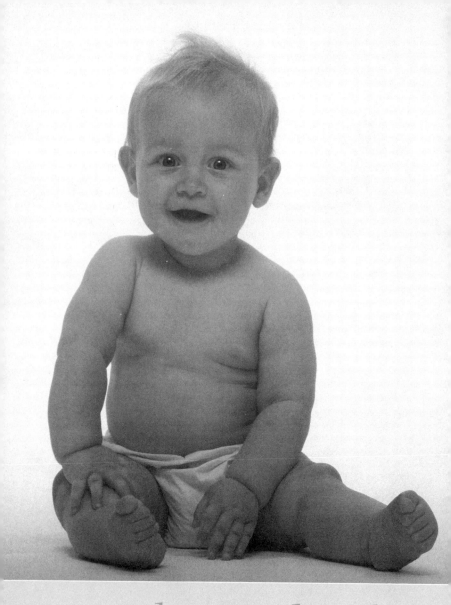

38 weeks and 6 days

8 days to go...

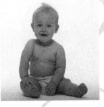

Baby names for girls and boys

Girls	Boys
Ula (Irish)	Ualtar (Irish)
Ulrica (German)	Ulmer (English)
Uma (Hindu)	Ulric (German)
Unity (English)	Urban (Latin)
Ursula (Latin)	Uri (Hebrew)

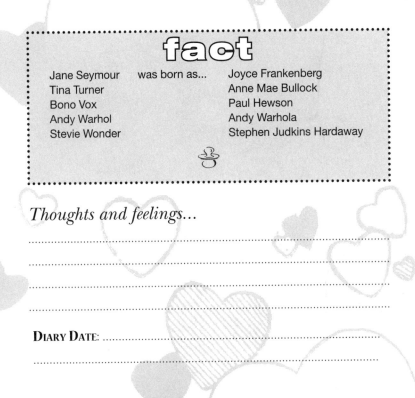

fact

Jane Seymour	was born as...	Joyce Frankenberg
Tina Turner		Anne Mae Bullock
Bono Vox		Paul Hewson
Andy Warhol		Andy Warhola
Stevie Wonder		Stephen Judkins Hardaway

Thoughts and feelings...

....

....

....

....

DIARY DATE: ....

....

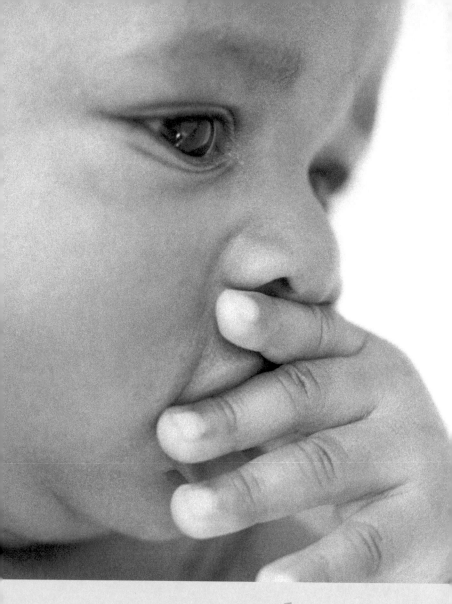

39 weeks

39 weeks

7 days to go...

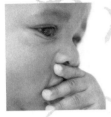

Your pregnancy

Your due date is still two weeks away, but for the last week, already, you have been within your 'calculated period'. This period covers five weeks: starting three weeks before your due date and ending two weeks after the calculated date. Your baby will be considered full term arriving anytime within this period. Don't travel too far away from home and make sure you always have the most important telephone numbers at hand.

Thoughts and feelings...

....

....

....

....

....

....

....

....

fact

After you have given birth you will instantly lose about 10–15lb (4.5–6.7kg). This is made up of baby, placenta, amniotic fluid and lochia. Although you are not back to your pre-pregnancy shape yet, you have certainly shed a heavy burden.

DIARY DATE: ....

....

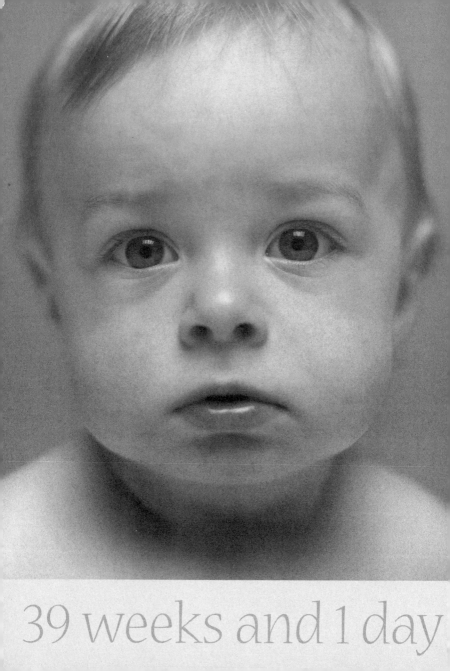

39 weeks and 1 day

6 days to go…

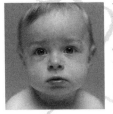

Did you know?

If you have teenage children and you announce the arrival of a new sibling, you may get a reaction ranging from horror to disgust. After all, your pregnancy advertizes the fact that you and your partner had sex—and this is almost incomprehensible to your teenage child. Plus, if you decide to breastfeed, baring your breasts may be met with a similar reaction. Teenagers have a lot to cope with, so try to be understanding about whatever they throw at you.

Thoughts and feelings…

....

....

....

....

....

....

....

....

remember

Having a new baby in the house can be a great form of sex education. Your teenage child will experience at first hand the never-ending responsibilities of caring for a small baby.

DIARY DATE: ....

....

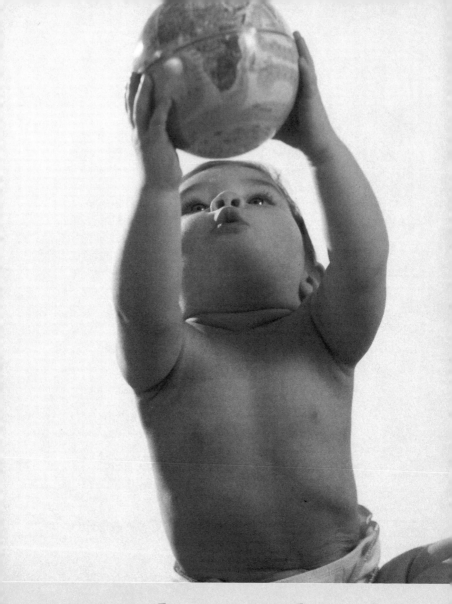

39 weeks and 2 days

5 days to go...

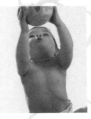

Giving birth

Six weeks after the birth of your baby you will see the doctor for a thorough check-up. Your blood pressure and urine will be checked again, and your stomach and breasts examined. You may be given an internal examination to check the size and position of your uterus. The doctor will make sure that any stitches have healed or are healing properly.

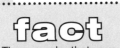

The eye color that your baby is born with will not necessarily be the color he finally has. It can change later in infancy or even childhood. This is due to the ongoing production of the hormone melanin, which influences eye color.

Thoughts and feelings...

....
....
....
....
....
....
....
....
....

DIARY DATE: ....
....

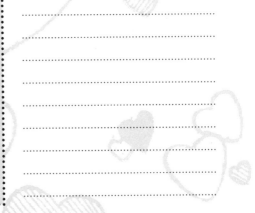

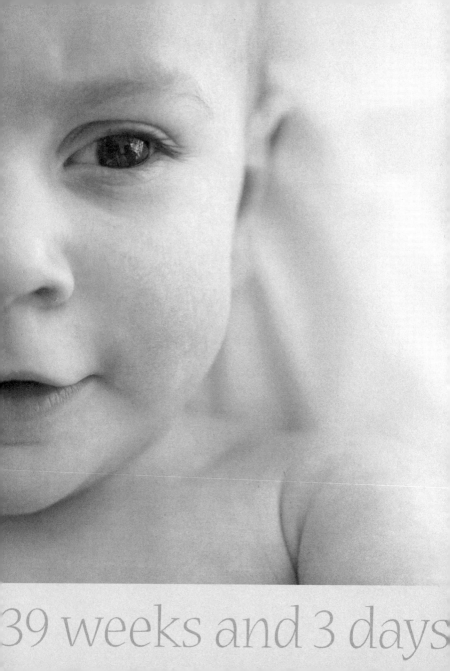

39 weeks and 3 days

4 days to go...

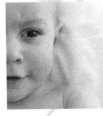

Health and fitness

In the weeks after giving birth you will probably notice differences in your hair; this is caused by hormonal changes. You may lose a lot of hair, or alternatively your hair may appear thicker than it was before pregnancy. Hair growth is generally stimulated during pregnancy. Use a mild shampoo and do not overbrush or dry hair vigorously with a towel. Allow it to dry naturally, if possible.

Thoughts and feelings...

....

....

....

....

....

....

....

....

Q&A

I'm having period pains after the delivery. Is this normal?

Slight cramps indicate your uterus is shrinking back to its normal size. Ten days after childbirth it will have contracted to one-twentieth of the size it was before labor. The cramps will probably stop a week or so after delivery, although breastfeeding can stimulate them again.

DIARY DATE: ....

....

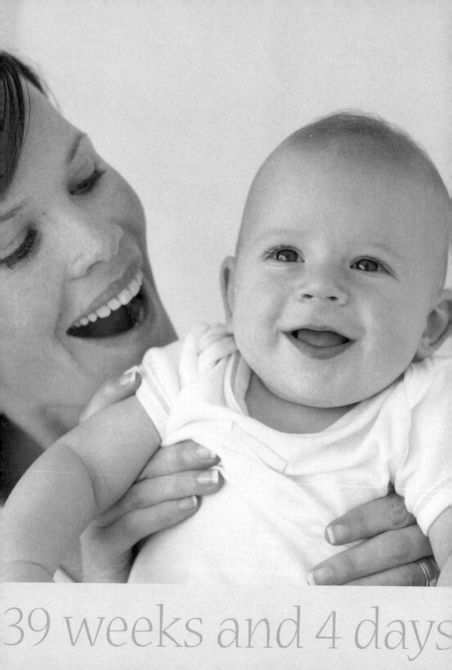

39 weeks and 4 days

3 days to go...

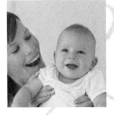

Baby's development

Everything is ready for the birth: the baby is hopefully in the right position. She is perfectly ready for life in the outside world now, but is still taking nourishment from the placenta. Only a small percentage of babies actually arrive exactly on the calculated due date, however, so you will have been in a state of anticipation for some time now. The baby is roughly 19¾in (50cm) in length.

Thoughts and feelings...

....

....

....

....

....

....

....

....

....

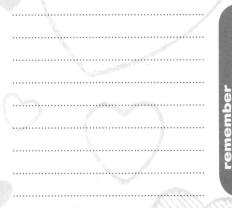

remember

If you want to use exercise to help get your body back in shape after giving birth, don't choose something that involves lots of extra paraphernalia. A baby, and everything that goes with it, will be enough to carry around to begin with.

DIARY DATE: ....

....

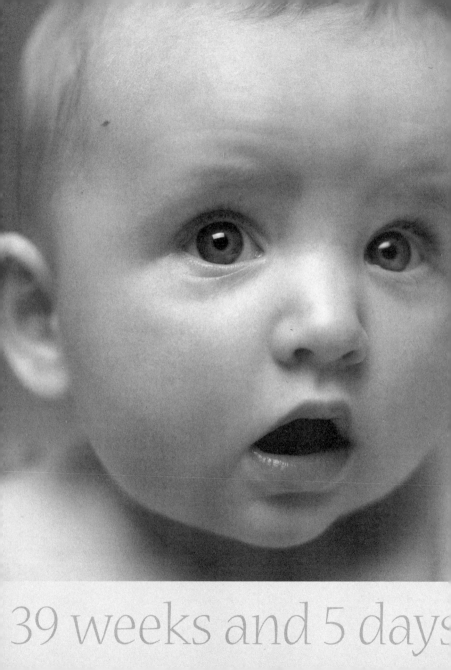

39 weeks and 5 days

2 days to go...

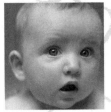

Did you know?

It's important to take time to introduce a new baby to your pet. Get your partner to take home some baby clothes so your pet can familiarize himself with her scent before they met. When you come in, greet your pet first, as he will be excited to see you after the separation. Then hold your baby and allow your pet to sniff around her gently, and get to know her.

"Any child can tell you that the sole purpose of a middle name is so he can tell when he's in trouble."

Dennis Fakes, author

WARNING

HOWEVER AFFECTIONATE AND TRUSTWORTHY YOU RATE YOUR PET, YOU SHOULD NEVER LEAVE YOUR NEW BABY UNATTENDED WITH AN ANIMAL— NOT EVEN FOR A MOMENT. YOU ALSO NEED TO BE VERY CAREFUL ABOUT HYGIENE.

Thoughts and feelings...

....
....
....
....
....
....
....

DIARY DATE: ....

....

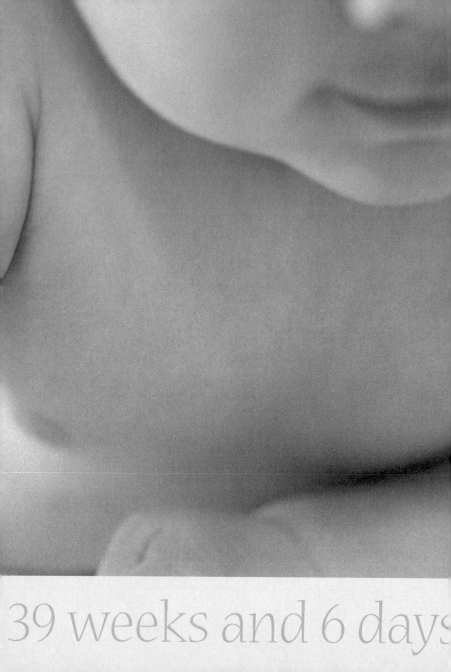

39 weeks and 6 days

1 day to go...

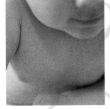

Baby names for girls and boys

Girls
Valerie (Latin)
Vanessa (Greek)
Vera (Slavic)
Verity (Latin)
Victoria (Latin)
Virginia (Latin)
Vita (Latin)

Boys
Vaughn (Welsh)
Victor (Latin)
Vincent (Latin)
Virgil (Latin)
Vivian (Latin)

Thoughts and feelings...

....
....
....
....
....
....
....
....
....
....

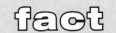

An old Irish naming tradition states that the first son should be named after the father's father, the second after the mother's father, the third after the father, and any additional sons (not so common today) after the father's brothers.

DIARY DATE: ....
....

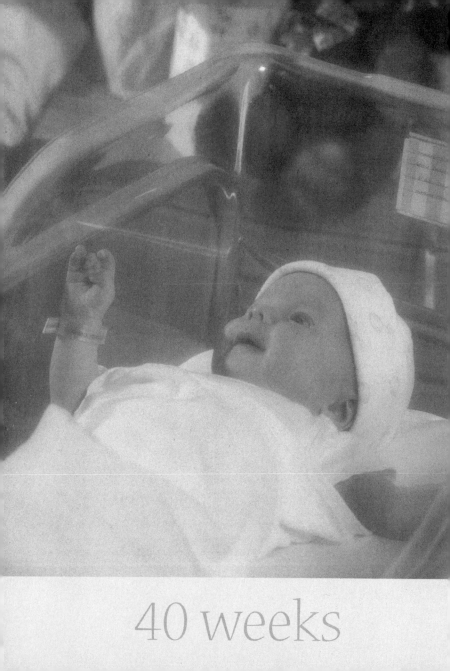

40 weeks

The big day!

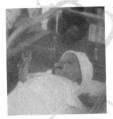

Your pregnancy

You have reached your calculated due date. Knowing that you really could give birth at any moment now could be affecting your mood in many different way. Perhaps you are restless and simply can't wait for things to move on; or possibly you are in a state of resignation and even tranquillity as you await the inevitable. The telephone is probably ringing more often than ever: family and friends all want to know how you are.

Thoughts and feelings...

....
....
....
....
....
....
....
....

DIARY DATE: ....

....

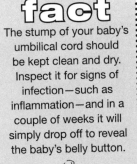

fact

The stump of your baby's umbilical cord should be kept clean and dry. Inspect it for signs of infection—such as inflammation—and in a couple of weeks it will simply drop off to reveal the baby's belly button.

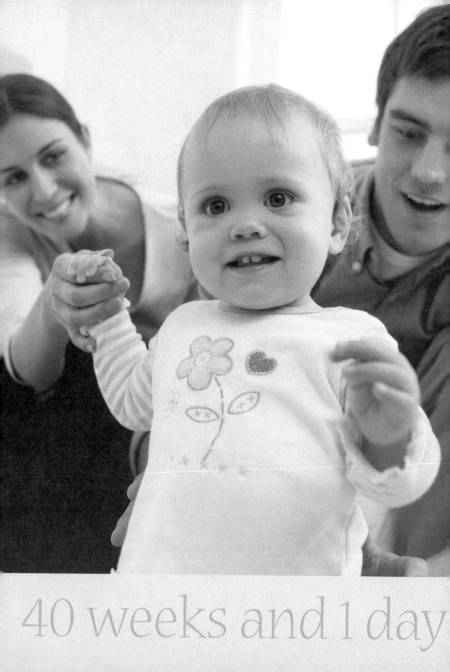

40 weeks and 1 day

1 day overdue...

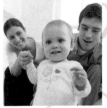

Did you know?

Many hospitals and health centers now run courses in baby massage. This is a great way for you to build contact with your baby and also to meet other new parents and hear their experiences of caring for a tiny baby. Massage can calm a distressed infant or simply relax your baby ready for a good night's sleep. It can be used to relieve stomach ache or constipation—and many babies suffer from these complaints.

Thoughts and feelings...

....

....

....

....

....

....

....

....

....

remember

Contact with other moms can bring you sociability and support. Look around for a baby and toddler group in your area, and if there isn't one, consider setting up a morning group yourself. A card on your pediatrician's bulletin board is a good place to start.

DIARY DATE: ....

....

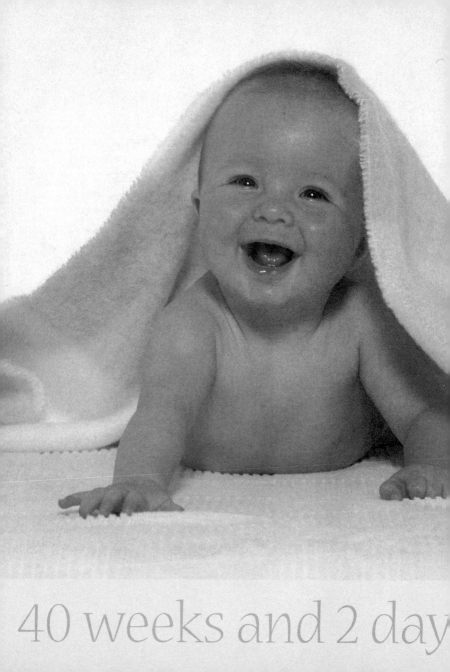

40 weeks and 2 day

2 days overdue...

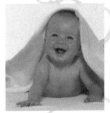

Giving birth

For the baby, as well as the mother, the birth is a challenging experience. Taken from the warm safety of the womb he is thrust under bright lights, blasted by cool air and unfamiliar noises and confronted by strange materials such as cloth, metal and plastic. Skin-to-skin contact with his mother is very important as your baby will recognize your smell and voice and immediately feel comforted.

Thoughts and feelings...

....

....

....

....

....

....

....

....

remember

Babies, both boys and girls, are often born with swollen genitals. This is due to the effects of your pregnancy hormones. Fathers who congratulate themselves on their well-endowed sons will notice a considerable reduction in size over time.

DIARY DATE: ....

....

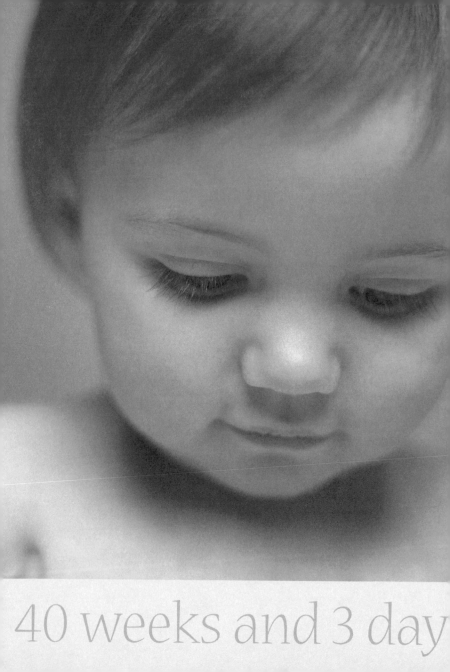

40 weeks and 3 day

3 days overdue...

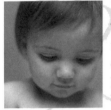

Health and fitness

Thyroid problems—either an over- or underactive thyroid—are fairly common after childbirth. Symptoms can mimic post-natal depression as well as leading to reduced milk supply, hair loss, heart palpitations and sleep disorders. They will also include either difficulty losing weight or rapid weight loss. Sometimes this is a temporary condition that will right itself; in other cases, medication can be prescribed to alleviate symptoms.

fact

If you suffer from temporary thyroid problems after childbirth you may be more susceptible to thyroid difficulties in later life. Talk to your doctor about having regular screening.

Thoughts and feelings...

....
....
....
....
....
....
....
....
....
....

DIARY DATE: ....
....

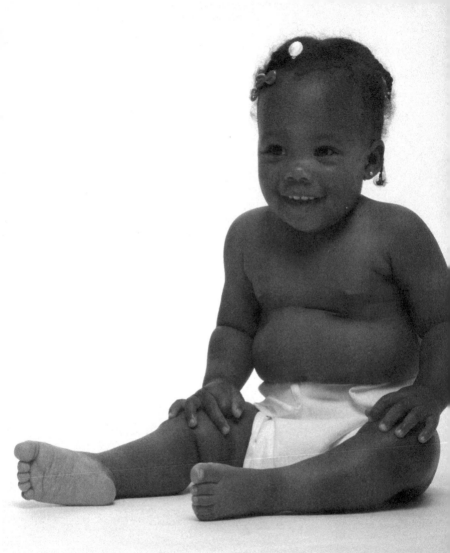

40 weeks and 4 day

0 weeks and 4 days

4 days overdue…

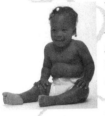

Baby's development

A beautiful moment is when your new baby grasps your finger. The Palmar, or grasping, reflex prompts her to close her fist around anything placed in her palm. She also has a rooting reflex: if you stroke her cheek she will turn her face to your touch and thus you can lead her to the breast or bottle. When startled she will automatically fling her limbs out and arch her back: you will want to protect her from this immediately.

Thoughts and feelings…

....
....
....
....
....
....
....
....

remember

The earlier your baby is born the more vernix and lanugo she will still have on her skin. Both will rub off over time, although you can help to remove vernix from her skin creases when she has her first bath.

DIARY DATE: ....
....

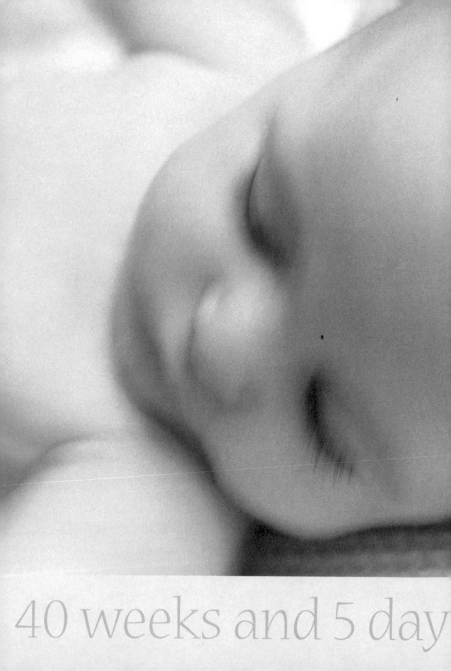

40 weeks and 5 day

5 days overdue...

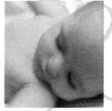

Did you know?

The term 'bonding' was first introduced in 1976 by two professors of pediatrics: Dr Marshall Klaus and Dr John Kennell. They claimed that close mother and infant contact was essential in the first 30 to 60 minutes after birth, for a strong bond to be built between the mother and her new baby. This can be upsetting to new mothers if, due to medical emergencies, they don't manage this contact: remember, you have a lifetime to bond with your child.

"I must say that the biggest lesson you can learn in life, or teach your children, is that life is not castles in the skies, happily ever after. The biggest lesson we have to give our children is truth."

Goldie Hawn, actress

Thoughts and feelings...

....

....

....

....

....

DIARY DATE: ....

....

remember

It is easy to lose faith in your parenting skills in the early days of caring for your new baby. It will take a little time for you to understand what he is trying to convey with his cries and squirms: but with patience you will work out a routine that suits you both.

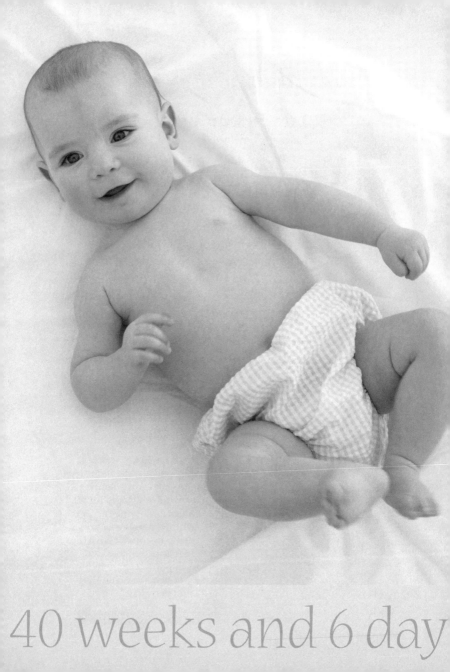

40 weeks and 6 day

6 days overdue...

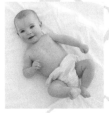

Baby names for girls and boys

Girls	**Boys**
Wallis (English)	Walter (German)
Wanda (German)	Warren (German)
Wendy (English)	Warwick (English)
Whitney (English)	Wesley (English)
Winifred (Welsh)	William (German)
	Winston (English)

Thoughts and feelings...

....

....

....

....

....

....

....

....

....

....

....

remember

If you already have children and would like to include them in choosing a name for their new sibling you could ask them to contribute ideas for a middle name. Of course, the more children you have the more middle names your new baby could end up with!

DIARY DATE: ....

....

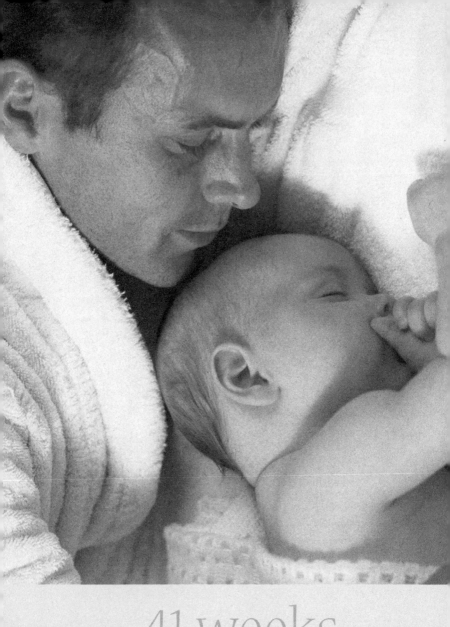

41 weeks

41 weeks

7 days overdue...

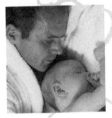

Your pregnancy

You may be keen to get your pre-pregnancy body back, but building an exercise regime into your day can be challenging in the first few weeks of looking after a baby. Wait until your six week check-up with the doctor before starting any major exercise, then start slowly—trying to find 20–30 minutes each day to get moving may still be a challenge.

Thoughts and feelings...

....

....

....

....

....

....

....

....

....

remember

If you include your baby in your exercise routine it may make it more realistic. Invest in a jogging buggy and take long walks or investigate mother and baby exercise classes at your hospital or community center.

DIARY DATE: ....

....

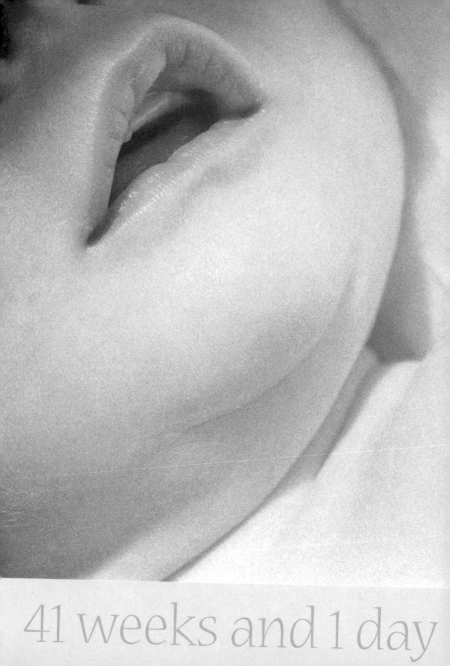

41 weeks and 1 day

8 days overdue...

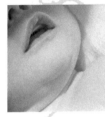

Did you know?

As your baby grows, your doctor or care provider will make you aware of various developmental targets she should reach and when. These are essentially screening tools, which, if a number are not reached, will draw your doctor's attention to potential problems. Remember the exact time frame for reaching these targets will vary from child to child: some get there sooner than others.

Thoughts and feelings...

....

....

....

....

....

....

....

....

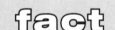

Sleep deprivation is responsible for a terrifying range of conditions from a reduced immune system to depression. Try to nap when your baby sleeps: and remember, your baby will learn to sleep through the night eventually.

DIARY DATE: ....

....

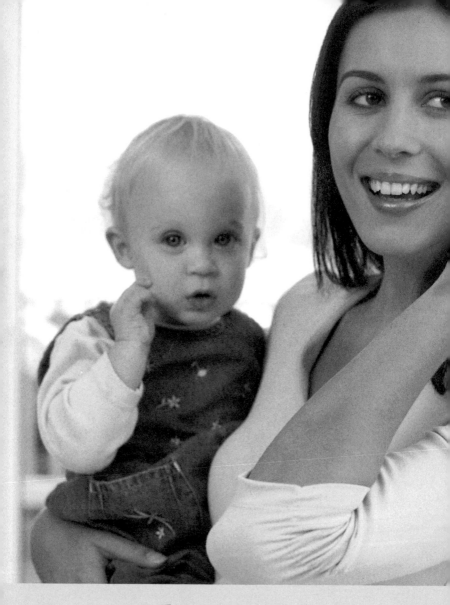

41 weeks and 2 days

9 days overdue...

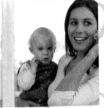

Giving birth

You may well find that your perineum, the area between your vagina and anus, has been bruised during childbirth. You may even have stitches after an episiotomy or tear. For some time afterwards the area may feel extremely tender, particularly when you are trying to relieve yourself. An ice pack may relieve soreness, or splashing with warm water or applying a hot-water bottle can also help.

Thoughts and feelings...

....
....
....
....
....
....
....
....

WARNING

IF YOU START TO DO TOO MUCH IN THE FIRST FEW WEEKS AFTER YOU HAVE GIVEN BIRTH, YOUR BODY WILL SOON LET YOU KNOW. IF YOUR LOCHIA FLOW BECOMES BRIGHT RED, THIS IS USUALLY AN INDICATION THAT YOU NEED TO TAKE A REST.

DIARY DATE: ....
....

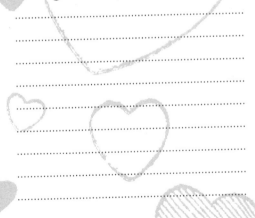

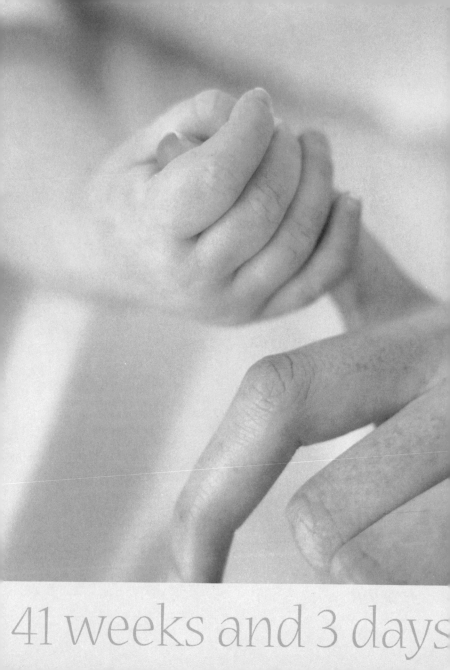

41 weeks and 3 days

10 days overdue...

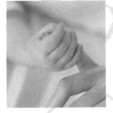

Health and fitness

Many new moms look forward to the time they can spend at home with their new baby—especially if they are planning to go back to work. However, these early days can be exhausting and it is likely that both friends and family will be keen to come and welcome your new arrival. You need to get used to your new life and may need time and space to do this. Politely put visitors off for a few weeks if you are feeling overwhelmed.

Thoughts and feelings...

....
....
....
....
....
....
....
....
....

Q&A

My wife and our baby are home now— when will things get back to normal?

Dads: it's time to accept that this is the new normal. The time you previously had for hobbies and relaxation may quickly get eaten up with caring for your baby and supporting your partner. Make sure you, too, get as much sleep as you can.

DIARY DATE: ....

....

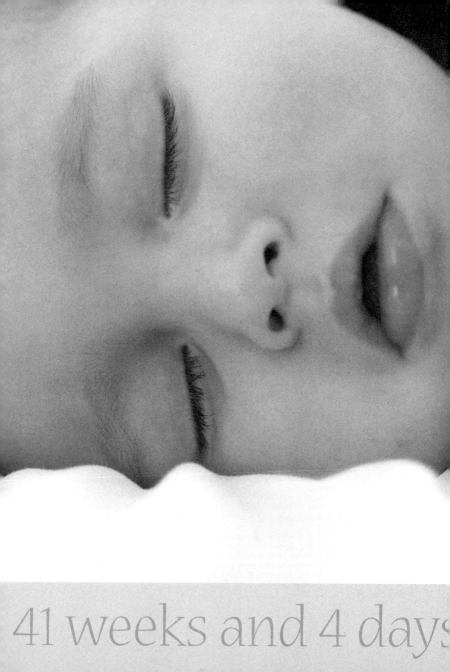

41 weeks and 4 days

11 days overdue...

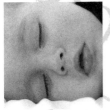

Baby's development

Most babies cry at some time, but if your baby cries on a regular basis for long periods of time (over two hours) and appears to be inconsolable, then perhaps she is suffering from colic. The crying fits are most likely to happen in the evening and she is likely to draw up her legs and screw up her fists as if she were in pain. Most colicky babies will improve by the time they are three months old, although some will still have bouts of colic after this.

Thoughts and feelings...

....

....

....

....

....

....

....

....

....

remember

Most babies will have periods of fretfulness, which will involve lengthy periods of crying. Overstimulation and growth spurts can be responsible, but you may simply have a sensitive baby who needs a little extra attention early in life.

DIARY DATE: ....

....

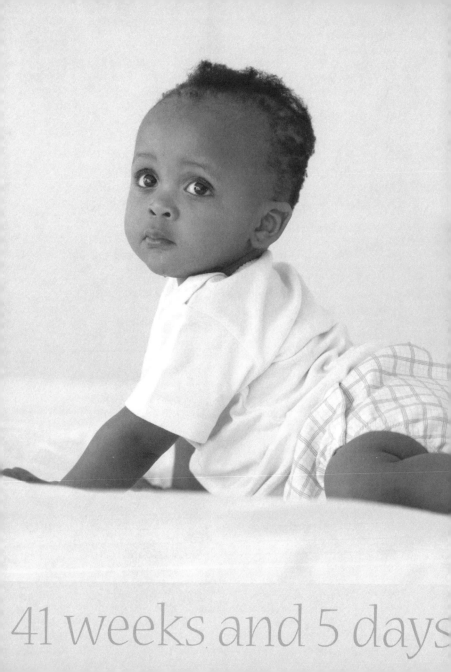

41 weeks and 5 days

12 days overdue...

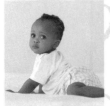

Did you know?

One of the hardest transitions after childbirth can be the return to the office. Try to ease the stress of separation—for both you and your baby—by going back gradually, perhaps on half-days or just a few days a week. Money and circumstances will influence your childcare choices, but other parents will be your best source of information regarding reliability and trustworthiness.

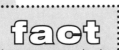

A nanny or au pair who comes to your home or lives with you is an easy, but expensive option for childcare. Alternatively, you may prefer your child to have a more sociable setting such as a daycare center.

"The best way to keep children home is to make the home atmosphere pleasant—and let the air out of the tires."

Dorothy Parker, poet and wit (1893–1967)

Thoughts and feelings...

....

....

....

....

....

DIARY DATE: ....

....

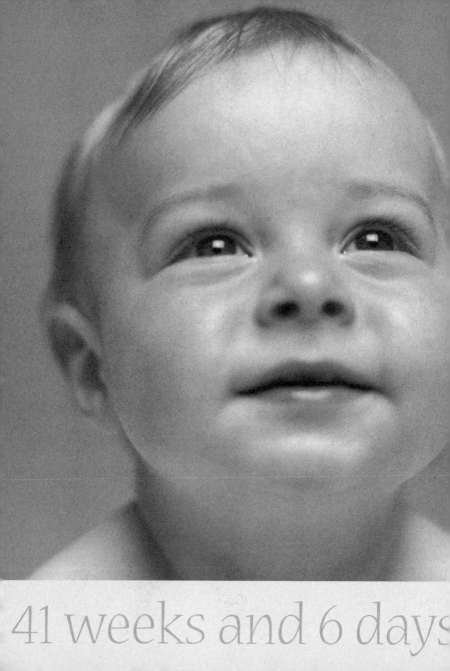

41 weeks and 6 days

13 days overdue...

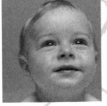

Baby names for girls and boys

Girls

Xandra (Spanish)
Xenia (Greek)
Yasmine (Arabic)
Yolanda (Greek)
Yvette (French)
Yvonne (French)
Zara (Hebrew)
Zoe (Greek)

Boys

Xavier (Spanish)
Yaakov (Hebrew)
Zachariah (Hebrew)
Zane (English)
Zeke (Hebrew)

Thoughts and feelings...

....
....
....
....
....
....
....
....
....

remember

Whether you are religious or not, the Bible and other books of faith are a great source of names for your children. The books of the Old Testament have provided names for generations of children worldwide.

DIARY DATE: ....
....

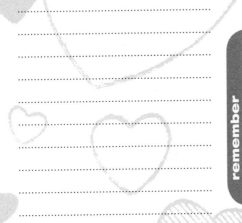

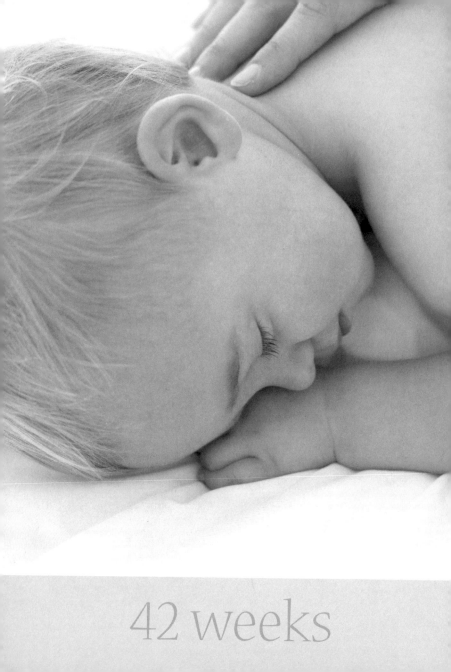

42 weeks

14 days overdue...

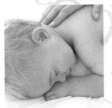

Your pregnancy

It really cannot be much longer now! If the baby doesn't give you some sign, you'll probably be induced. If you haven't already had it, you will certainly have an appointment with your care provider this week for them to assess your condition and the progress of your baby. Whatever happens next... Good luck!

remember

If you start to overshoot your due date by more than a week, this could be an indication that you were muddled over the date of your last period when calculating your due date. The size of the baby may also be a clue as to whether this has happened.

Thoughts and feelings...

....

....

....

....

....

....

28	Week 1						
	1	2	3	4	5	6	7

First day of your last period

Week 2						
8	9	10	11	12	13	14

Ovulation, impregnation

| january | 1 | 2 | 3 | 4 | 5 | 6 | 7 | 8 | 9 | 10 | 11 | 12 | 13 | 14 | 15 | 16 |
| october | 8 | 9 | 10 | 11 | 12 | 13 | 14 | 15 | 16 | 17 | 18 | 19 | 20 | 21 | 22 | 23 |

| february | 1 | 2 | 3 | 4 | 5 | 6 | 7 | 8 | 9 | 10 | 11 | 12 | 13 | 14 | 15 | 16 |
| november | 8 | 9 | 10 | 11 | 12 | 13 | 14 | 15 | 16 | 17 | 18 | 19 | 20 | 21 | 22 | 23 |

| march | 1 | 2 | 3 | 4 | 5 | 6 | 7 | 8 | 9 | 10 | 11 | 12 | 13 | 14 | 15 | 16 |
| december | 6 | 7 | 8 | 9 | 10 | 11 | 12 | 13 | 14 | 15 | 16 | 17 | 18 | 19 | 20 | 21 |

| april | 1 | 2 | 3 | 4 | 5 | 6 | 7 | 8 | 9 | 10 | 11 | 12 | 13 | 14 | 15 | 16 |
| january | 6 | 7 | 8 | 9 | 10 | 11 | 12 | 13 | 14 | 15 | 16 | 17 | 18 | 19 | 20 | 21 |

| may | 1 | 2 | 3 | 4 | 5 | 6 | 7 | 8 | 9 | 10 | 11 | 12 | 13 | 14 | 15 | 16 |
| february | 5 | 6 | 7 | 8 | 9 | 10 | 11 | 12 | 13 | 14 | 15 | 16 | 17 | 18 | 19 | 20 |

| june | 1 | 2 | 3 | 4 | 5 | 6 | 7 | 8 | 9 | 10 | 11 | 12 | 13 | 14 | 15 | 16 |
| march | 8 | 9 | 10 | 11 | 12 | 13 | 14 | 15 | 16 | 17 | 18 | 19 | 20 | 21 | 22 | 23 |

| july | 1 | 2 | 3 | 4 | 5 | 6 | 7 | 8 | 9 | 10 | 11 | 12 | 13 | 14 | 15 | 16 |
| april | 7 | 8 | 9 | 10 | 11 | 12 | 13 | 14 | 15 | 16 | 17 | 18 | 19 | 20 | 21 | 22 |

| august | 1 | 2 | 3 | 4 | 5 | 6 | 7 | 8 | 9 | 10 | 11 | 12 | 13 | 14 | 15 | 16 |
| may | 8 | 9 | 10 | 11 | 12 | 13 | 14 | 15 | 16 | 17 | 18 | 19 | 20 | 21 | 22 | 23 |

| september | 1 | 2 | 3 | 4 | 5 | 6 | 7 | 8 | 9 | 10 | 11 | 12 | 13 | 14 | 15 | 16 |
| june | 8 | 9 | 10 | 11 | 12 | 13 | 14 | 15 | 16 | 17 | 18 | 19 | 20 | 21 | 22 | 23 |

| october | 1 | 2 | 3 | 4 | 5 | 6 | 7 | 8 | 9 | 10 | 11 | 12 | 13 | 14 | 15 | 16 |
| july | 8 | 9 | 10 | 11 | 12 | 13 | 14 | 15 | 16 | 17 | 18 | 19 | 20 | 21 | 22 | 23 |

| november | 1 | 2 | 3 | 4 | 5 | 6 | 7 | 8 | 9 | 10 | 11 | 12 | 13 | 14 | 15 | 16 |
| august | 8 | 9 | 10 | 11 | 12 | 13 | 14 | 15 | 16 | 17 | 18 | 19 | 20 | 21 | 22 | 23 |

| december | 1 | 2 | 3 | 4 | 5 | 6 | 7 | 8 | 9 | 10 | 11 | 12 | 13 | 14 | 15 | 16 |
| september | 7 | 8 | 9 | 10 | 11 | 12 | 13 | 14 | 15 | 16 | 17 | 18 | 19 | 20 | 21 | 22 |

15	16	17	18	19	20	21

22	23	24	25	26	27	28

1

4 weeks pregnant

| 17 | 18 | 19 | 20 | 21 | 22 | 23 | 24 | 25 | 26 | 27 | 28 | 29 | 30 | 31 | january |
| 24 | 25 | 26 | 27 | 28 | 29 | 30 | 31 | 1 | 2 | 3 | 4 | 5 | 6 | 7 | november |

| 17 | 18 | 19 | 20 | 21 | 22 | 23 | 24 | 25 | 26 | 27 | 28 | | | | february |
| 24 | 25 | 26 | 27 | 28 | 29 | 30 | 1 | 2 | 3 | 4 | 5 | | | | december |

| 17 | 18 | 19 | 20 | 21 | 22 | 23 | 24 | 25 | 26 | 27 | 28 | 29 | 30 | 31 | march |
| 22 | 23 | 24 | 25 | 26 | 27 | 28 | 29 | 30 | 31 | 1 | 2 | 3 | 4 | 5 | january |

| 17 | 18 | 19 | 20 | 21 | 22 | 23 | 24 | 25 | 26 | 27 | 28 | 29 | 30 | | april |
| 22 | 23 | 24 | 25 | 26 | 27 | 28 | 29 | 30 | 31 | 1 | 2 | 3 | 4 | | february |

| 17 | 18 | 19 | 20 | 21 | 22 | 23 | 24 | 25 | 26 | 27 | 28 | 29 | 30 | 31 | may |
| 21 | 22 | 23 | 24 | 25 | 26 | 27 | 28 | 1 | 2 | 3 | 4 | 5 | 6 | 7 | march |

| 17 | 18 | 19 | 20 | 21 | 22 | 23 | 24 | 25 | 26 | 27 | 28 | 29 | 30 | | june |
| 24 | 25 | 26 | 27 | 28 | 29 | 30 | 31 | 1 | 2 | 3 | 4 | 5 | 6 | | april |

| 17 | 18 | 19 | 20 | 21 | 22 | 23 | 24 | 25 | 26 | 27 | 28 | 29 | 30 | 31 | july |
| 23 | 24 | 25 | 26 | 27 | 28 | 29 | 30 | 1 | 2 | 3 | 4 | 5 | 6 | 7 | may |

| 17 | 18 | 19 | 20 | 21 | 22 | 23 | 24 | 25 | 26 | 27 | 28 | 29 | 30 | 31 | august |
| 24 | 25 | 26 | 27 | 28 | 29 | 30 | 31 | 1 | 2 | 3 | 4 | 5 | 6 | 7 | june |

| 17 | 18 | 19 | 20 | 21 | 22 | 23 | 24 | 25 | 26 | 27 | 28 | 29 | 30 | | september |
| 24 | 25 | 26 | 27 | 28 | 29 | 30 | 1 | 2 | 3 | 4 | 5 | 6 | 7 | | july |

| 17 | 18 | 19 | 20 | 21 | 22 | 23 | 24 | 25 | 26 | 27 | 28 | 29 | 30 | 31 | october |
| 24 | 25 | 26 | 27 | 28 | 29 | 30 | 31 | 1 | 2 | 3 | 4 | 5 | 6 | 7 | august |

| 17 | 18 | 19 | 20 | 21 | 22 | 23 | 24 | 25 | 26 | 27 | 28 | 29 | 30 | | november |
| 24 | 25 | 26 | 27 | 28 | 29 | 30 | 31 | 1 | 2 | 3 | 4 | 5 | 6 | | september |

| 17 | 18 | 19 | 20 | 21 | 22 | 23 | 24 | 25 | 26 | 27 | 28 | 29 | 30 | 31 | december |
| 23 | 24 | 25 | 26 | 27 | 28 | 29 | 30 | 1 | 2 | 3 | 4 | 5 | 6 | 7 | october |

Notes...

Notes…

Notes...

Notes...

Notes…

Notes...

Notes...

Notes...

Notes...